SERIES ON NURSING ADMINISTRATION

EDITORIAL BOARD

SERIES ON NURSING ADMINISTRATION

VOLUME 3   **MARCH 1992**

The Delivery of Quality Health Care

Editor
Marion Johnson, RN, PhD
Assistant Professor
College of Nursing
The University of Iowa
Iowa City, Iowa

Chair of the Board
Joanne Comi McCloskey, RN, PhD, FAAN
Professor
Nursing Service Administration
College of Nursing
The University of Iowa
Iowa City, Iowa

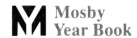
Mosby
Year Book

St. Louis   Baltimore   Boston   Chicago   London   Philadelphia   Sydney   Toronto

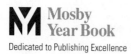
Mosby
Year Book
Dedicated to Publishing Excellence

Editor: N. Darlene Como
Editorial Assistant: Barbara M. Carroll
Project Manager: Peggy Fagen

International Standard Book Number 0-8016-6524-8

92 93 94 95 96   GW/MV   9 8 7 6 5 4 3 2 1

Contents

Contributors

Peter I. Buerhaus, RN, PhD
Assistant Professor
College of Nursing
The University of Iowa
Iowa City, IA

M. Patricia Donahue, RN, PhD, FAAN
Associate Professor
College of Nursing
The University of Iowa
Iowa City, IA

Diane L. Gardner, RN, PhD
Assistant Professor
College of Nursing
The University of Iowa
Iowa City, IA

Charlene Harrington, RN, PhD
Associate Director
Institute for Health and Aging
School of Nursing
University of California
San Francisco, CA

Ada Jacox, RN, PhD, FAAN
Professor, Independence Foundation
  Chair in Health Policy
School of Nursing
Johns Hopkins University
Baltimore, MD

Marion Johnson, RN, PhD
Assistant Professor
College of Nursing
The University of Iowa
Iowa City, IA

Ellen Marszalek-Gaucher, RN, MPH
Senior Associate Director
University of Michigan Medical Center
Ann Arbor, MI

Joanne Comi McCloskey, RN, PhD,
  FAAN
Professor
College of Nursing
The University of Iowa
Iowa City, IA

Marilyn T. Molen, RN, PhD
Dean of Nursing
Metropolitan State University
St. Paul, MN

Mychelle M. Mowry, RN, MN
Director, Nursing Information Systems
Cedars-Sinai Medical Center
Los Angeles, CA

Barbara Pillar, RN, PhD
Nurse Scientist Administrator
Nursing Systems Branch
National Center for Nursing Research
National Institutes of Health
Bethesda, MD

Peggy Reiley, RN, MSN, MPH
Director of Quality Assurance and
  Development
Beth Israel Hospital
Boston, MA

Anne Rooney, RN, MA
Director, Accreditation Programs for
  Hospice and Home Care
Joint Commission on Accreditation of
  Healthcare Organizations
Oakbrook Terrace, IL

Patricia Schroeder, RN, MSN
Nursing Quality Consultant
President, Quality Care Concepts, Inc.
Editor, Journal of Nursing Quality
  Assurance
Editor, Nursing Quality Connection
Thiensville, WI

Cheryl B. Stetler, RN, PhD
Director of Clinical Practice
Hartford Hospital
Hartford, CT

Karen Zander, RN, MS, CS
The Center for Nursing Case
  Management, Inc.
South Natick, MA

Volume IV
Planned Contents

Theme—Doing More With No More:
Economic Myths and Realities

Publisher's Note

Nurse administrators play a vital role in establishing and maintaining environments that support high-quality, cost-effective nursing care in the varied settings in which nurses practice today. The issues and trends affecting health care delivery and nursing, in particular, are increasingly complex and dynamic. More than ever before, nurse administrators need a convenient, ongoing forum for communicating ideas, concerns, experiences, insights, and strategies with their peers. The *Series on Nursing Administration* provides just such a forum.

Mosby–Year Book, Inc. is proud to serve as the new publisher of the *Series on Nursing Administration*. Our commitment to nurses and nursing is stronger than ever, and we are pleased to bring this valuable information resource to nurse administrators. We hope you will be challenged and enlightened by each volume of the series.

Series Preface

Today's nurse executive needs to stay current in many rapidly changing areas of health care. To meet this demand, the *Series on Nursing Administration* is designed to give nursing administrators new information on current and emerging issues. Developed and managed at the University of Iowa College of Nursing and published by Mosby–Year Book, Inc., it is a quality resource for nurse executives, faculty who teach nursing administration, and students in nursing administration programs. Each year a new volume addresses the most recent issues in the complex and dynamic discipline of nursing administration. Thus a subscription to the series will keep readers on the forefront of knowledge and practice.

Every nurse executive relates upward to higher corporate management levels; outward to colleagues in other settings, to professional groups, to the community, and to consumers; and downward to nursing and ancillary personnel and to clients within the hospital. To stay current with developments on all these levels, the nurse executive reads journals and newsletters, attends continuing education programs, and participates in short-term executive management courses. The most effective method, however, is the sharing of concerns, experiences, and insights with peers. The Mosby–Year Book *Series on Nursing Administration* formalizes the process of sharing among experts with similar concerns. In every chapter of each volume of the series, expert authors share their experiences and ideas on particular emerging issues. Busy nurse executives can conveniently and cost effectively keep their knowledge current on a variety of topics by reading this series.

Nursing administration faculty can use the series not only to keep their teaching alive but also to keep current and timely themselves. Most nursing administration programs have one or more courses that address issues in nursing management. Because these issues undergo rapid change, faculty need a flexible approach to teaching this content. This series offers the instructor maximum flexibility in selecting issues for discussion to fit the needs of a particular class. An instructor teaching a nursing management issues course can use the series as a course text. Students introduced to this series will find it a resource with ongoing value. Faculty teaching undergraduate level administration courses may also use the series to supplement an introductory text on management and leadership.

This series is unique in that it is the first annual series devoted to issues in nursing administration. To ensure that it covers current issues and provides up-to-date information, the series employs a unique publication process involving four groups: a series editor, an editorial board, the authors, and the publisher.

The editor of Volumes I to IV of the series is Marion Johnson, RN, PhD, an assistant professor at the University of Iowa. She has a rich practice base in nursing administration and currently teaches nursing administration at the master's level. Her background, interests, and writing skills make her eminently qualified for the job of series editor.

The editorial board consists of faculty teaching in the nursing administration program at the University of Iowa and selected nurse administrators associated with the program. The board meets three or four times a year with the series editor, helps identify the emerging issues and prospective authors, and assists the editor with manuscript review. The University of Iowa's growing program in nursing administration, including study at the doctoral level, makes this an ideal setting to support this publication.

The authors are distinguished nurse administrators and educators chosen for their expertise in particular areas. While authors have the freedom to pursue an issue as they choose, each is encouraged to address the state of knowledge, future directions, and controversial questions surrounding the issue and to propose one or more options for resolution.

The publisher of the series, beginning with this volume, is Mosby–Year Book, Inc. Volumes I and II, initially published by Addison-Wesley, are now also available from Mosby. Mosby's senior nursing editor, Darlene Como, has provided encouragement and assistance with continued development of the series. An annual series is unique in the literature of nursing administration, and we are fortunate that Mosby–Year Book is committed to its success.

All of us involved in this series believe that it will benefit those who teach and practice nursing administration as well the entire nursing profession and, most importantly, the patients we serve. We welcome your comments and suggestions.

Joanne Comi McCloskey, RN, PhD, FAAN
Chairperson, Editorial Board, Volumes I-IV

Introduction

Nurse administrators are facing increased pressure to demonstrate the quality of nursing services provided in their organizations. Health care consumers and payers are demanding answers to questions about the quality, effectiveness, and cost of available health care services. Access to quality health care has become a societal, organizational, and professional problem as the number of uninsured increases. Health care professionals are facing demands to identify and quantify the effects of their interventions and treatments. Without doubt, the quality of health care services provided in the United States will be a major concern for consumers, payers, and providers during the next decade.

This volume is devoted to issues that surround the delivery of quality health care and in particular to those factors that affect quality nursing care. The book is comprised of three sections focusing on the following topics: the evolution of the meaning and measurement of quality, quality assurance applications in specific settings and with specific methodologies, and the environmental and professional developments that impact the quality of nursing care.

Each chapter develops a specific topic and its related issues, but the reader will note a number of themes related to the establishment and assessment of quality recurring throughout the book. First is the changing terminology: quality improvement, total quality management, effectiveness, appropriateness, and cost-effective care are examples of these changes. Second are value shifts that are being reflected in policy changes in health care. Third is the increased role of government in forcing the definition and measurement of quality. Fourth is the consensus that economic factors will continue to have a substantial impact on how quality will be defined during the next decades. Last, but of significant concern for nursing, is the need to develop measures of quality, particularly in the arena of patient outcomes. While these themes recur throughout the book, they are presented from differing perspectives by each of the authors.

During the preparation of this volume, the publisher of the *Series on Nursing Administration* changed. Readers familiar with the first two volumes in the series will note a number of format changes in the current volume. These changes are a result of recommendations from Darlene Como, our editor at Mosby–Year Book, Inc. and the editorial board for the *Series.* My sincere thanks to all involved for assisting with these changes. Also, I owe a debt of gratitude to all of the authors who so willingly updated their chapters for this volume. It is hoped that this work will not be in vain and that the volume will generate questions, raise issues, and offer insight and advice for nurse administrators as they struggle with defining and measuring quality in their organizations.

Marion Johnson
Editor

The Evolution of Quality

The evolution taking place in the definition and measurement of quality health care is explored from a number of perspectives in this section of the text. Previous efforts directed toward the assurance of health care quality and the problems inherent in these efforts are described by a number of the authors. Current issues and trends in quality assurance, quality improvement, and quality monitoring are presented. This content provides a background for considering the quality applications and the influence of environmental changes presented in the following sections.

The answer to the question "What is quality health care?" is formed by values: personal, professional, and societal. The chapter by Donahue focuses on these values and how they influence the definition of health care quality. Problems faced by nursing in ensuring quality in an evolving health care system dominated by economic concerns are presented, and nurses are challenged to clarify what future nursing practice should be. After this discussion, economic constraints and the implications of market competition in health care are explored in the chapter by Buerhaus. The implications of market competition for nursing care quality are explicated, including the need for innovation and risk taking on the part of nurse leaders and administrators.

The movement toward interdisciplinary collaboration for quality improvement programs, as well as the changes necessary for success, are discussed in a brief but cogent chapter by Schroeder. Problems and issues related to the development and use of measures of quality are discussed by Gardner. Included in Gardner's chapter is a discussion of prominent measures of nursing care categorized according to the concepts measured: nursing functions, nursing competency, and outcomes of nursing care.

The last chapter, by Johnson and McCloskey, presents an overview of current governmental and private efforts that are under way to ensure effective health care relative to quality, outcomes, and cost. Also presented are a number of issues that must be resolved for nurses to assume their desired role in these national endeavors. The reader will find a number of the programs described in this chapter referred to throughout the volume.

CHAPTER 1

Health Care Values and Quality

M. Patricia Donahue

The rapid economic and technologic changes taking place in health care are forcing a reevaluation of the values that shape the health care system and a reexamination of how quality care is defined. As these processes move forward, nursing can have a pivotal role in determining the health care system of the future and the role of nursing in this system. To do so will require vision, creativity, and the willingness to make decisions about opposing values and to take the risks inherent in these decisions. Nurse administrators are in a position to help create a quality nursing and health care system for tomorrow.

I foresee continued conflict between the "bureaucrats" and the "healers" primarily because we, the people who cheer on both, are so utterly confused about the social role of health care as we switch back and forth from the status of cool and calculating potential patients to the state of being aching and frightened actual patients. No one, of course, adds more to this confusion than economists who, at least while in a state of good health, sincerely seem to believe that individuals who are acutely ill, or their anxious relatives, can be viewed as ordinary "consumers" (Bulger, 1988, pp. xv-xvi).

As the twenty-first century looms on the horizon, a multitude of questions regarding the complexion and complexity of American health care

The University of Iowa, Iowa City, IA 52242.

Series on Nursing Administration – Volume III, 1992

are being raised. Foremost among them are those questions that are posed in an attempt (1) to retain traditional values in a society in which technology almost reigns supreme, (2) to guide American health policy toward greater social harmony, (3) to alleviate social dilemmas created by competing or changing sets of values, or both, (4) to confront the realities of current health care economics, and (5) to ensure quality health care. Unfortunately there will be no easy answers or solutions, because the issue of health care touches the innermost core of human existence. The majority of persons regard health care as something extremely personal and meaningful and worry that assistance will not be available when needed. They wonder how and by whom decisions will be made in the face of limited resources, who will receive lifesaving organs when not all can, whether the best care possible will be rendered in all situations, whether health care will be available to all, and where financial resources will be obtained to ensure the provision of quality care.

The literature currently abounds with books and articles in which authors attempt to come to grips with a rapidly changing health care system that mandates new and creative approaches to problems. Philosophers, ethicists, physicians, sociologists, theologians, and economists, as well as professionals from other disciplines, attempt to provide insights and solutions to dilemmas that arise in a complicated, expensive, and "high-tech" health care arena. It is thus apparent that awesome forces within society continue to shape the evolution of health care, health care values, and quality of care. It is equally apparent that there still is some doubt about the value of technology and uncertainty about the specific factors that determine high-quality care. Is quality care to be defined ultimately in terms of technologic sophistication? Is the best care always what is technically possible? Is more always better than less?

In the context of these happenings, the future of nursing practice must be contemplated. Such was the intent of a national forum, "Nursing Practice in the 21st Century," a collaborative effort of the American Nurses Foundation (ANF) and the Annenberg Center for Health Sciences. Two purposes were identified for exploration at this conference (ANF, 1988, p. 1):

1. The role of nursing in the twenty-first century, a role expected to expand and change as the general population and community-based health care services increase
2. The development of options through which nursing and the public and private sectors can collaborate to ensure that appropriate nursing services are available in the home and community settings now and into the future

At this forum, nurses and representatives of corporations, government, philanthropy, the media, and other health care interest groups contemplated the future of nursing practice. The assumption was that the best options for immediate and future actions on issues facing nursing and the health care system would come from a diversity of views. As the forum unfolded, a significant theme emerged from *all* participants — that nurses may be (are) uniquely prepared to meet the health care and social challenges of the future (ANF, 1988, p. 4):

> nursing embodies the values, concerns, and interests most appropriate for responding to the complexities of health care today and in the future. Society will benefit as nurses integrate their humanistic and caring values into the highly technological health care marketplace and diversify their services within existing and expanded settings.

The voices from nursing's past echo in these statements. Health care may be changing, but the traditional values of nursing are still relevant. What remains to be done, therefore, is to effectively balance the humanistic, traditional nursing values with a highly technologic, highly specialized delivery system that is being forced to operate under cost containment. Such is the challenge of the next century! Such is the challenge for nursing! Such is the challenge for all who are involved in the delivery of health care.

TECHNOLOGY, VALUES, AND HEALTH CARE

The increasing dominance of technology in health care has had a direct effect on the delivery of health care services and has influenced the value system that determines the services to be delivered and the manner in which they will be delivered.

Reflections on Technology

There is no doubt that the health care system is in rapid flux. This does not imply that health care has ever been static or that similar problems have not been encountered previously. What is potentially different is the rise of technologic intervention to a significant and powerful position in the health care industry. Technology, however, must not be thought of *only* in terms of its physical manifestations, such as those devices, machines, and artifacts that can extend human capabilities and displace persons as the focus of interest. Technology also includes the procedures (control techniques and systems) used to operate, monitor, and evaluate the devices. Essentially, it "can be understood as concerned with the national arrangement of devices and procedures for the achievement of definite, measurable, useful, and relatively immediate outcomes" (Barger-Lux & Heaney, 1986, p. 1313).

During the last 30 to 40 years, technology has become a primary and dominant force in all facets and at all levels of health care. Frequent references are now made to the "technical fix," "technological dominance," the "technical order," and the "technological imperative in health care" (Barger-Lux & Heaney, 1986; Cassell, 1974; Crawshaw, 1983; Fuchs, 1968). The meaning of these terms is clear—technologic intervention continues at an escalating pace in many facets of our lives. Significant decisions about human life are being made on the basis of available technology.

The health care industry has not been immune to a mentality of bigger, better, and faster. Health care agencies clamor for increased budgets to enable purchase of the latest in technology as rapidly as it becomes available. Hospitals and other agencies have learned very quickly which equipment, which diseases, and which clinical units generate the greatest income and provide the greatest profit. Diagnostic and treatment procedures often are compensated to a greater degree by third-party payers than are traditional clinical skills and preventive measures. Unfortunately, the technology is not only expensive but also at times irrelevant. A number of authors even pose the view that too much technology is used too often in situations in which either benefit *has not been proved* or *is short-lived* (Barger-Lux & Heaney, 1986; Bulger, 1988; Jennett, 1986; Perkoff, 1986). For example, statistics demonstrate that approximately 50% of patients who are admitted to intensive care units (ICUs) are either too sick or too well to benefit from this care. Even more crucial is the use of therapeutic interventions against patients' desires. The focus of care, too often, is not the patient but the application of devices and procedures. Thus the continued and increased use of technology for diagnosis and treatment is not without its problems as new issues are generated and must be resolved.

Has this proliferation of technology in health care become a double-edged sword? Certainly those who have analyzed the impact of technology have debated *potential* benefit versus *potential* harm. (Perhaps effectiveness research will debate *real* benefit versus *real* harm.) A list of factors can be generated to support each edge of the sword. Perceived and stated benefits seem, however, to reside more in the philosophic realm and, at times, to be less clearly defined. Technology is viewed as a force for good and evidence of the human being's inquiring mind and creative spirit. Technology allows for a wider range of options in treatment decisions, thereby allowing freedom of choice. Perhaps the most vivid benefits relate to technologies that provide for "miracle cures" and "delays of death" under the bleakest of circumstances. In addition, increased job opportunities become available in a variety of settings and marketplaces, new companies are developed, and hospitals compete with one another for the most expensive, complicated, and well-equipped specialized units possible. The competitive spirit in this instance is viewed as a positive outcome. Finally, technology can facilitate more rapid and accurate diagnoses and provide health care practitioners with more time. All these benefits, as well as others, supposedly contribute to the health and well-being of the society and directly or indirectly enhance health care. When all is said and done, a belief pervades that technology in combination with science can resolve almost everything.

The other edge of the sword concerns perceived and stated harm. Much of this dialogue deals with decision making in the areas of economics, allocation and use of resources, and ethics, all of which are influenced by the fear or risk of legal action. Barger-Lux and Heaney believe that the primary reason for opposition to the technologic imperative is that technologic solutions to health problems are "an inadequate response to complex human situations that involve life and death, health, and bodily integrity" (1986, p. 1315). They specify that the dignity and worth of the human being are being threatened by the valuing of things over people (p. 1318):

> When technology dominates, the operating purpose of health care can be death prevention rather than the preservation and restoration of functional capacity and responsible autonomy. It is as though both caregivers and patients become extensions of the devices and procedures that occupy center stage. Things that are important in human terms—what we have termed the issues of human value—can become quite obscured. Also, the technological imperative is associated with a kind of health care—doing everything possible for individuals already in the system—that is showing itself to be financially burdensome, that restricts creation of a dignified and appropriate "floor" of the services for all, and that too often opposes the wishes and legitimate interest of patients themselves.

What is being discussed here are the conflicting and competing values that are shaping modern health care. Bulger's depiction (1988) of this conflict is quite vivid as he refers to competing values of healing and bureaucracy. The healing side typifies the "micro" or "clinical" ethic of health care concerned with the moral imperatives used at the patient's bedside; the bureaucracy side typifies the "macro" or "social" ethic of health care concerned with the allocation of society's scarce resources to competing ends. Of primary concern is the advent of the overall effect of a depersonalization of care and patient displacement, which have become a problem and a reality. Even dying has moved from the moral to the technical order. Technologic success has facilitated a societal mythology that moral things can be made technical, that human events such as birth and death can be altered by technology. This altering of fate creates an illusion in American society that "fate can be defeated" (Cassell, 1974, p. 32).

There is no doubt that moral and ethical problems related to technology will have long-lasting effects that are regarded by many as harmful to society. Few would deny that benefit has resulted and will result from technology. Concerned voices, however, are being raised to protest the rapid erosion of the humanistic aspects and humanistic values in health care. Within this context, the question of benefit *and* cost to patients must be strongly considered. Equally important is the reduction in the care-giving work force, fueled by the high cost of technology. Health care personnel, as well as patients, are being displaced. What all of this ultimately means remains to be seen. One cannot dismiss, however, that shifts in values have occurred that have effectively diminished the movement toward health care as a right with equal access for all.

There is no doubt that shrinkage in reach and accessibility is already occurring in the health care system (Curtin & Zurlage, 1991). Local hospitals have been forced to close while clinics and city and county medical centers are being inundated by those who have been socially and economically "caught in the middle."

Value Transition in Health Care

Positions regarding the relevance, influence, and impact of values in health care currently proliferate in the literature. Various statements are consistently made regarding the shifting of values in health care, the changing values in the health care delivery system, competing sets of values in health care, and conflict in and collision of values. Whatever phraseology is used, the meaning is clear—values that drive health care and health care delivery are in a state of flux. In addition, not all agree on what values should dominate in dealing with the health and well-being of individuals within the society. A conceptualization of health care can mean many different things to many different people and may, in fact, rest with an individual's perception of personal gain. Various forces such as politics and economics also serve either to replace operating values with new values or to generate a hierarchy of values in health care. Certainly technology has created a mind set that almost anything is possible in dealing with human illnesses, which may further influence value choices. Pellegrino speaks eloquently to this idea (1979, p. 11):

> When all things are possible, then we must decide which ones we shall have. What we choose, however, unerringly reveals what we value and that, in turn, peels back the layer of protection covering what we think we are and what we think humans are for.

Perhaps "value restandardization" is a better label for the technologic effect that results in change in the value structures of the work place: "For example, the values of honesty, loyalty, and integrity are still found in the workers' hierarchy of values, but their relative positions and what *constitutes* each of them may have been (needs to be?) revised considerably" (Curtin, 1986, p. 7). In other words, long-lasting values have not been discarded but may occupy a different position in the hierarchy or have decreased priority in the scheme of things.

It is not always easy to determine which values are currently prominent and affect quality in the health care system. Rapid change in combination with almost insurmountable forces frequently serves to obscure the value issues. Even more distressing is the idea that health care workers, including nurses, function under value sets that they do not understand, do not agree with, or feel powerless to change. Although values motivate and guide their actions, these may not be the values they choose to express. For example, nurses may be forced to function in systems in which high priority is placed on economic constraint and efficient use of personnel. Nurses' values related to quality patient care, as well as respect for patients' rights, safety, and best interests, may thus be compromised. Therein lies another difficulty related to values—that values operate at different levels, frequently at the same time. Individual values, microvalues (family, institution), and macrovalues (society) may all be operating at the same time and may indeed be in conflict both within levels and between levels (Wright, 1987). What must be emphasized is that nursing and nurses function in the real world. Consequently, those values that have served nursing well in the past but may no longer be relevant must be sifted out; those values that continue to be relevant should be kept. Still other values may need to be altered in some way, for example, shifted or reprioritized. The traditional values of quality care and patient advocacy, however, need to be constantly reaffirmed but may need to be restructured in light of social reality.

Few would disagree with the statement that "a value is a quality having intrinsic worth for a society, and American society's dominant values significantly influence all decisions concerning health care policies" (MacPherson, 1987, p. 3). Yet MacPherson's analysis (1987, 1991) of the current situation regarding health care policy and values might give rise to some disagreement even though it is consistent with much of the available dialogue on the subject. Her assessment is that the dominant American values of individualism, competition, and inequality shape American health care policy. Consequently, the values of collectivism and cooperation, which would ensure equal access to health care resources, are inoperable. MacPherson makes a plea for change but recognizes that changing values is not easy. She clearly identifies, however, those of the cultural and political elite who shape and guard values that reflect and support their interests as government officials, private foundation representatives, corporate executives, and blue-ribbon presidential commission members.

Individualism, competition, cost containment, efficiency, and technology are the values that currently are driving health care policy and health care systems while also affecting quality nursing care both positively and negatively.

THE QUESTION OF QUALITY

Quality . . . you know what it is, yet you don't know what it is. But that's self-contradictory. But some things *are* better than others, that is, they have more quality. But when you try to say what quality is, apart from the things that have it, it all goes *poof*! There's nothing to talk about. But if you can't say what Quality is, how do you know what it is, or how do you know it even exists? (Pirsig, 1974, p. 163).

With the current emphasis on the quality of health care and its measurement, one tends to believe that quality is a new and different issue that we are now forced to encounter. Yet questions concerning quality have all been raised before and studied to a greater or lesser degree: What is quality health care? What constitutes quality care? How can quality of care be measured? How can the quality of care be improved? What is the cost for quality care? What is disheartening are the tendencies to ignore what has been discovered in the past about quality care and the considerable knowledge and experience available regarding its measurement. Much emphasis still focuses on the determination of a definition of quality of care and the development of measurement techniques (Brook, Williams, & Avery, 1976; Menninger, 1975; Wyszewianski, 1988). This in and of itself is not destructive but serves to foster the status quo rather than *improvement* in the quality of care.

It is obvious that problems surround the issue of quality of care. There are certainly claims that no one can really define what quality care is, let alone measure it. Perhaps this claim is proposed because of the difficulty involved with its assessment. Perhaps it is proposed because of the diversity of opinions and perceptions regarding its makeup. For example, some patients define quality of care in terms of highly sophisticated and technologic services in which many and frequent diagnostic tests are performed (Barger-Lux & Heaney, 1986). A physician may define quality on the basis of knowledge and execution of skills, whereas a nurse may define it in terms of a holistic view of the patient. In some instances, hospital mortality rates have become synonymous with quality of care! Thus personal and professional perceptions of quality, as well as environmental, political, organizational, and economic forces, influence identification of the specific components of quality care.

Historically, the interest in and understanding of quality of care have waxed and waned. The notion can be traced as far back as ancient civilizations in which very descriptive punishments were inflicted on the physician who failed to heal the patient. Wyszewianski (1988) provides a historical account of pioneers in quality of care assessment, thereby vividly demonstrating that this area not only was written about but also was studied as far back as the early 1900s: "As Donabedian has pointed out, advances in the early 1930s and in the mid-1950s laid down 'the foundations of almost all the major approaches to quality assessment.' To these two periods must be added the late 1960s, when Donabedian's own seminal contributions established the basic vocabulary and concepts we now use in talking about quality of care" (Wyszewianski, 1988, p. 13).

What becomes clear in Wyszewianski's provocative discussion is that the reasons for concern about quality vary, such as in the late 1960s when health care expenditures were rapidly escalating. At times, overprovision of services to the patient has been at issue; at other times, the possibility of underprovision of services has been at issue. It is apparent that the current interest has been dramatically affected by cost containment and fueled by the advent of diagnosis-related groups (DRGs) and market competition. The historical focus on the preservation of the status quo left no incentive for improvement in quality; it is hoped that improvement will be fostered through the current emphasis on total quality management.

Quality of care assessment involves a number of variables, including the elucidation of the benefits and harms, actual or potential, that result from care; the efficacy and efficiency of treatments and programs; the technical quality of care, as well as the quality of other aspects of care such as the interpersonal component; and the influence of amenities (comfort, appeal, and so forth) within the health care system. All these have an impact on nursing and its ability to render quality care and effectively act as the advocate for the patient. The mandate for nursing rests with the determination of what constitutes *quality nursing care* and *how it can be practiced*, given the constraints that currently are operating in the health care system.

A relevant document, "Features of High Quality, Cost-Effective Nursing Care Delivery Systems of the Future," was prepared by the National Commission on Nursing Implementation Project (NCNIP, 1988). It is certainly a seminal work that represents a compilation of data from a variety of sources. The intent of this work was the identification of a model that would (1) provide for the creation of quality and cost-effective nursing care delivery systems and (2) offer guidance for the development of successful future nursing care delivery systems. The members of this Commission readily recognized that health care is rapidly changing, that nursing functions in all types of systems, and that nurses have the most sustained contact with patients and are a primary force in the movement toward wellness. Each of these facts lends credence to the statement that "nursing services are pivotal in health care delivery and have a valuable contribution to make to its design" (NCNIP, 1988, p. 1).

Ten features of high quality, cost-effective nursing care delivery systems were organized by the Commission into four clusters (NCNIP, 1988, p. 2):

1. *Delivery-related characteristics*: those that affect the circumstances under which quality nursing services are provided, for example, working relationships among nurses, physicians, and the other members of the health care team
2. *Evaluation-related characteristics*: those that affect the quality control aspects of nursing care delivery
3. *Marketing-related characteristics*: those that affect the demand for nursing services

4. *Policy-related characteristics*: those that affect nursing's ability to influence overall policies in organizations where nurses provide services

Although one could question whether all aspects of this document could feasibly be incorporated into a health care delivery system, its beauty lies in the identification of strategies for change that are flexible enough to be useful at all levels and in all types of organizations in which nursing functions. Even more exciting is the emphasis on nursing accountability to consumers and their care, to organizations in which nursing services are provided, and for fiscal resources for nursing practice. This element of accountability may serve as the catalyst to resolve two issues: the realization of "nurse as patient advocate" and a decision concerning what realistically can be achieved in patient care. Mere talk about patient advocacy is not enough; how to be a patient advocate under the constraints of DRGs and various prepaid health insurance plans must be learned and must be practical. In the final analysis, however, "the major stumbling block in efforts to improve quality of care is still the difficulty in successfully changing clinicians' practice patterns" (Wyszewianski, 1988, p. 19). The Commission document represents one more attempt to specify characteristics or features of quality nursing care, yet also suggests alternative practice patterns.

In any discussion of quality of care it *must be understood* that its delivery is not the exclusive province of nursing. It is the shared responsibility of all health care professionals and must involve a public that participates in the control and improvement of its own health. All too often, nursing tends to assume responsibility for whatever ails the health care delivery system rather than engaging in effective dialogue and activity that will promote interdisciplinary responsibility for quality assurance. The public must be taught to assume responsibility, particularly in respect to health protection; it must be taught that costly medical technology is no substitute for continuous monitoring of its own health and health practices. Finally, a balance must be achieved between the quality of technical care and the quality of the art-of-care: "Technical care refers to the adequacy of the diagnostic and therapeutic processes; and art-of-care relates to the milieu, manner, and behavior of the provider in delivering care to and communicating with the patient" (Brook et al., 1976, p. 6). According to these authors, efforts at increasing quality typically have gone into improving the technical aspects of care. The irony in this practice is that improvements in the art-of-care may effect greater changes in health. It is thus time that researchers measure the art-of-care side of the scale to determine the overall impact on health improvement created versus that created by improved technical aspects of care. Nurses could and should be the trend setters in this area of research inasmuch as the art of nursing is almost synonymous with the art-of-care. Perhaps the real secret to quality of care is best expressed in the following statement:

"One of the essential qualities of the clinician is interest in humanity, for the secret of the care of the patient is in caring for the patient" (Peabody, 1927, p. 878).

THE CONTINUING CHALLENGE

One point of view that can be applied to quality control is expressed as follows (Seay, Vladeck, Kramer, Gould, & McCormack, 1986, p. 257):

> There is a school of thought among experiential, if not academic, managers that events which confront an institution can be divided into two categories: those you can control and those you cannot. The conventional wisdom further states that the important thing is to recognize the difference between the two, and to avoid spending undue time, energy, and resources attempting to control the uncontrollable. Rather, one should concentrate one's efforts toward having a measurable impact on those things over which control can be exerted.

The challenge of the future for nursing and nurses is to shape a reality-based practice world rather than a dangerous fantasy world. The fact remains that there are forces and influences in the health care delivery system over which nursing has little control. There are, however, areas over which nursing can influence the direction of health care delivery and create a force whereby this influence can be achieved. Nursing must realize that it has the capacity to shape its future and its practice arena. The key ingredient, however, to such an accomplishment is the need for nursing first to clarify what kind of practice it wants and then to take the initiative to make it happen. Insight is essential here, as well as a collaborative effort among nurses. No one nurse or group of nurses can effect the needed changes; all nurses must work together, keeping in mind what is needed for nursing *as a whole* to progress.

The profession of nursing must always reach toward the ideal, with the understanding that reality is what dictates practice. Nursing of the future will require more than good managing. It will require new and creative ways to deal with the diverse needs of the society being served. It will require making decisions about opposing values and forces that are plaguing the health care system. Styles (1988, p. 61) referred to these as "points" and "counterpoints":

Points	Counterpoints
Quality	Cost
Focus	Expand
Nursing values	Marketplace values
Shaping	Reacting
Independence	Integration
Health services	Social/human services
Acute care	Wellness care
Look inward	Look outward
Opportunity	Disaster

TABLE 1-1   Health Care Delivery Paradigm Shift

Medical/cure model	Chronicity/continuity/community
Disease-based (deficits)	Need-based (attributes)
High technology	Low technology
High specialization	Low specialization (paraprofessionals,
Rigid boundaries	volunteers)
Fragmentation, duplication	Soft boundaries
	Integrated
	Multidisciplinary consultation
Episodic reimbursement	Case-based reimbursement
(keep beds full)	(keep beds empty)
Revenue	Cost-savings models
Patient-centered	Centered on family and social support
Hierarchy of decision	Interactional: Collaborative decisions
Appeals to authority	Empowers consumer/family decisions
Power of protected information	Power in shared information
Short-term planning	Long-range planning
Crisis management	Outcome-oriented
Process-oriented	

Reprinted with permission from S. Ryan, "Transition from institutional to home and ambulatory care." In *Nursing Practice in the 21st Century*, Copyright 1988 by the American Nurses' Foundation, Kansas City, MO.

She stated that it could be argued that they are not dichotomous nor mutually exclusive and that the key to the future might be to render them compatible. Even more striking is her comment that "where we cannot reconcile, we must choose" (p. 61). Consistent with this discussion is Ryan's paradigm (Table 1-1), which compares the current model of health care delivery that is disease-based or deficit-based with a needed future model that is more needs-based or attribute-based. Ryan's model of the future is based on the life-style and chronicity needs evidenced in the 1980s (1988, p. 44).

CONCLUSION

The next few years can be an interesting period in which to live and work. It can be an exciting period of growth, achievement, and great satisfaction if nursing identifies what it cannot change and where it has no choices. At the same time, nursing must change those things that can be changed to ensure quality patient care and to exercise choice with thoughtful deliberation. Nurse administrators and nurse executives are in a unique position to foster an environment in which they can work collaboratively with clinical nurses to create viable, humanistic, efficient, and effective practice settings that will embody the traditional nursing values of caring, compassion, quality, and advocacy. As Ralph Waldo

Emerson noted, "This time, like all times, is a very good one, if we but know what to do with it."

REFERENCES

American Nurses' Foundation. (1988). *Nursing practice in the 21st century*. Kansas City, MO: Author.

Barger-Lux, M. J., & Heaney, R. P. (1986). For better and worse: The technological imperative in health care. *Social Science Medicine, 22*, 1313-1320.

Brook, R. H., Williams, K. N., & Avery, A. D. (1976, November 21-22). Quality assurance in the 20th century: Will it lead to improved health care in the 21st? *Proceedings of the Boston University Conference on Quality Assurance in Hospitals* (pp. 1-43), Boston: Boston University.

Bulger, R. J. (1988). *Technology, bureaucracy, and healing in America*. Iowa City: The University of Iowa Press.

Cassell, E. J. (1974). Dying in a technological society. *Hastings Center Studies, 2*, 31-36.

Crawshaw, R. (1983). Technical zeal or therapeutic purpose—How to decide? *Journal of the American Medical Association, 250*, 1857-1859.

Curtin, L. L. (1986). Sister Angelique "blows the whistle . . . ." *Nursing Management, 17*, 7-8.

Curtin, L. L. & Zurlage, C. (1991). Cornerstone of healthcare in the nineties: Forging a framework of excellence—A report of a landmark conference. *Nursing Management, 22*, 32-43.

Fuchs, V. R. (1968). The growing demand for medical care. *New England Journal of Medicine, 279*, 190-195.

Jennett, B. (1986). *High technology medicine: Benefits and burdens*. New York: Oxford University Press.

MacPherson, K. I. (1987). Health care policy, values, and nursing. *Advances in Nursing Science, 9*, 1-11.

MacPherson, K. I. (1991). Health care policy, values, and nursing. In M. J. Ward & S. A. Price (Eds.), *Issues in Nursing Administration* (pp. 91-101). St. Louis: Mosby–Year Book, Inc.

Menninger, W. W. (1975). Caring as part of health care quality. *Journal of the American Medical Association, 234*, 836-837.

National Commission on Nursing Implementation Project. (1988). *Features of high quality, cost-effective nursing care delivery systems of the future*. Milwaukee, WI: Author.

Peabody, W. (1927). The care of the patient. *Journal of the American Medical Association, 88*, 877-882.

Pellegrino, E. D. (1979). *Humanism and the physician*. Knoxville: The University of Tennessee Press.

Perkoff, G. T. (1986). Ethical aspects of the physician surplus: Implications for family practice. *Journal of Family Practice, 22*, 455-460.

Pirsig, R. M. (1974). *Zen and the art of motorcycle maintenance*. New York: Bantam Books.

Ryan, S. (1988). Transition from institutional to home and ambulatory care. In American Nurses' Foundation (Ed.), *Nursing practice in the 21st century* (pp. 41-45). Kansas City, MO: American Nurses' Foundation.

Seay, J. D., Vladeck, B., Kramer, P., Gould, P., & McCormack, J. (1986). Holding fast to the good: The future of the voluntary hospital. *Inquiry, 23*, 253-260.

Styles, M. (1988). Summary and recommendations. In American Nurses' Foundation (Ed.), *Nursing practice in the 21st century* (pp. 53-62). Kansas City, MO: American Nurses' Foundation.

Wright, R. A. (1987). *Human values in health care: The practice of ethics*. New York: McGraw-Hill.

Wyszewianski, L. (1988). Quality of care: Past achievements and future challenges. *Inquiry, 25*, 13-22.

CHAPTER 2

Nursing, Competition, and Quality

Peter I. Buerhaus

A competitive market requires that organizations attend both to costs and to quality in the production of goods or services, or both. A number of recent developments in health care financing are shifting the supply side of the market toward a competitive market, but changes also are needed on the demand side for true market competition to emerge. Market competition in health care has the potential for affecting both the practice of nursing and the provision of nursing services. To advance nursing in a competitive environment, nursing leaders will need to be innovators and risk takers.

Perhaps the most important policy shift in health care that emerged during the 1980s was the adoption of traditional market forces as a legitimate strategy to achieve greater efficiency in the production of health care services. This shift represents a movement away from, if not an explicit rejection of, the regulatory strategy that dominated the health care system in the 1970s. Reliance on the regulatory approach, such as voluntary planning, certificate of need, hospital rate review, and profes-

Partially supported by a Division of Nursing Advanced Nurse Education Grant (1D23NU00812).
The University of Iowa, Iowa City, IA 52242.

Series on Nursing Administration — Volume III, 1992

sional standards peer review, not only failed to constrain annual increases in health care costs but inadequately protected the public from incompetent providers and overuse of medical care such as unnecessary surgery. Despite public admonitions that regulations were required to ensure high-quality health care, in reality providers (especially hospitals), professionals (especially physicians), and insurers (especially Blue Cross) favored only the weakest mechanisms to assure quality while strongly and consistently supporting other regulations that advanced their economic self-interests and enabled them to create monopolistic positions in their respective health care markets (Feldstein, 1988b). As monopolists, these suppliers determined the type and amount of health care provided, controlled the kind of facilities in which services have been provided, and obtained regulatory barriers to protect themselves from others seeking to enter their markets and threaten their excessive earnings. Had health care been governed less by regulation and more by traditional market forces, the chances of the development of monopolistic power would have been reduced, and providers and professionals would have been forced to compete on the basis of price, quality, and the extent to which they provided services that were more responsive to consumers' preferences rather than to their own.

Now that traditional market forces, which rest on the principles of economic competition, have become a legitimate strategy to achieve socially desirable outcomes in health care,[1] many policy makers and analysts have seriously questioned what will happen to the quality of health care services. Not surprisingly, physicians, who would have much to lose if forced to compete to a greater extent on the basis of cost, have decried that a competitively oriented health care system inevitably will lead to a deterioration of quality and result in a massive reorganization of the system (Relman, 1983). Nurses too have expressed skepticism concerning the compatibility of competition and high-quality health care (Boyar, 1985). Regardless of one's point of view on the desirability of competition, the direction of change is clear, and its course is indicated by the policy debate that has shifted away from the question, "Will competition play an important role in health care?" to one that asks, "How can we make competition work to rearrange the incentives of providers and purchasers so that health care is produced more efficiently and costs are controlled without endangering quality?"

This chapter attempts to provide a framework for addressing some of the issues that underpin the success of the emerging competitive strategy in health care. By first reviewing the traditional market forces that have long governed economic activity in our nation's economy and next examining some of the problems that need to be resolved before competition can fully take hold, it will then be possible to assess if and how competition is likely to affect the quality of health care and the practice of nursing. This approach also will be useful to anticipate and discuss some issues that may affect the nursing profession and that might not otherwise be considered in this volume. A final purpose is to stimulate more nurses, especially those in management and research roles, to become more active in developing quality assessment methods that both incorporate and capitalize on nursing's unique contributions and yet are consistent with the realities of an increasingly competitive health care marketplace.

A REVIEW OF MARKET COMPETITION

Throughout the 1980s, nurses heard about the health care system's adoption of traditional market forces primarily in terms that created the expectation that competition would help control health care costs. Although no one suggested that health care was being or should be stripped of all regulations, a strong belief was shared by many health policy formulators, by federal and state governments, and by academia that market competition should exert a greater role in guiding economic decisions (Brown, 1988; Havighurst, 1983). Belief in the benefits derived from market competition spans political boundaries as well: beginning in the Carter administration and continuing with the Reagan and Bush administrations, explicit government policies (helped by changing economic conditions) have resulted in substantial "deregulation" of the railroad, trucking, telecommunications, and financial services industries. Today these industries are far more competitive than in the past. The process of deregulating an industry, however, does not happen overnight and does not occur without causing substantial stress and uncertainty as firms in the industry being deregulated, as well as those who are employed by them, learn how to respond to different economic incentives.

As market competition becomes a more dominant force in the economic organization of health care, one way for nurses to anticipate what lies ahead for the health care industry and for the nursing profession is to examine what has occurred in the industries that have been deregulated and then to draw analogies to health care. Although this would be a useful and entertaining approach, it carries the risk of making misleading predictions, because each of the aforementioned industries is unique, and analogies with the health care industry probably would fail to adequately incorporate its peculiarities and highly personal nature. An alternative approach is to examine the incentives that underpin traditional market forces and then make logical inferences as to what might happen in health care and the possible effects on those who make their living in this industry. An important advantage of this approach is that it keeps a sharp focus on the economic interests and the interrelationship among health care providers, professionals, employers, and employees and how they are likely to change. An understanding of the principles of economic competition requires the ability to anticipate the consequences of allowing traditional market forces to operate in health care; thus these forces are reviewed next, followed by a discussion of some of the problems that need to be overcome before competition can more fully evolve in health care.

Principles of Market Competition

In a market characterized by price competition, firms (suppliers) have an incentive to produce their goods or services at minimum cost so that they can be priced at a level at which consumers are willing to purchase them. If priced too high, many buyers would be unwilling to purchase the good or service and would shop around until they found either the same good or a substitute at a lower price.[2] Knowing that a substantial part of buyers' purchasing decisions is based on the price of the good or service, firms have an incentive to keep prices low enough so that they can sell their products and still make a reasonable profit.

To keep product prices low, firms must produce goods at or near minimum cost. For this to occur, firms must be the right size (neither too big nor too small) to take advantage of any economies of scale (receive quantity discounts on purchases of commodities, obtain cost savings from automating production or certain managerial functions, access capital at favorable interest rates). Firms also must be innovative in the way they combine the capital, labor, and technology used to produce their goods, and they must buy these factors of production at the lowest possible price. If a firm fails to keep production costs low, others who have been quicker and more successful to innovate and to take advantage of new technology or changes in capital and labor will find ways to produce their goods at a lower cost. Consequently, the firm that produces at lower cost will be in a position to offer its products at a price below the prevailing market price and therefore sell more of its products and earn greater profits. Unless the competing firm matches or lowers the price of the good produced by its competitor, it will not sell as much as before and will earn smaller profits. Eventually, firms whose costs are higher may go out of business. Thus, in a competitive market, suppliers have an incentive to minimize production costs so that they can price their products competitively, earn profits, and stay in business.

Although price plays a crucial role, it is not the only determinant of consumers' demand or willingness to make purchases of goods and services. Other factors include the amount of consumers' income, unique preferences or tastes, the price of other related goods, and whether consumers actually want or need the good at any particular time. Although firms can do nothing to change consumers' income in order to influence them to buy more of their products, market research enables them to discover what products consumers want and how much they are willing to spend. Knowing the tastes and preferences of consumers, a firm then attempts to produce and sell the desired product before its competitors. Microcomputer firms, for example, constantly respond to consumers' preferences by developing and offering computers that are easier to operate, faster, and have a greater number of unique and useful applications. To ensure their consumers' awareness of their products, as well as to positively influence their tastes and desire for them, firms promote their products through advertising. Advertising also provides consumers with valuable information on the price of the product and its unique noneconomic characteristics, which helps consumers to form an impression about the product's quality and distinguish it from other products on the market.

A firm can charge higher prices for higher-quality products in part because production costs may be higher and some consumers are willing to make trade-offs between price and quality. That is, some consumers prefer a more expensive good and will pay a higher price in exchange for what they perceive is higher quality. Aware that, in addition to price, consumers consider the product's quality in making purchasing decisions, firms cannot be indifferent about buyers' perception of quality. If consumers perceive that the product's quality is low, then they may be unwilling to purchase it unless, of course, the price is also very low. Thus firms have strong incentives not only to be innovative so that they can minimize production costs and price their products competitively but also to be responsive to consumers' preferences and perceptions of their product's quality.

In a competitive marketplace consumers or buyers (the demand side of the market) are given choices in the goods and services they can purchase. Influenced by their level of income, tastes, and preferences, as well as the amount of information on the product, consumers consider the trade-off between price and quality and purchase the products that are most satisfying. By purchasing certain products of a defined quality and price and not others, consumers tell suppliers whether their products are priced "right" and meet expectations in quality and availability. With such information, suppliers make necessary modifications to their products so that consumers will be more satisfied with them and more likely to make future purchases. In this important way, suppliers and demanders in competitive markets are in touch with each other, but satisfying the consumer is the only sure way that firms can sell their products and earn profits. As the saying goes, "The consumer is king."

Assumptions Underlying Competition

Economists and health policy analysts have long debated whether competition can realistically become a way of organizing economic activity in health care. The debate has centered largely on the conditions that are assumed necessary for competition to work. Fuchs (1988) identified these conditions as (1) a large number of buyers and sellers, no one of whom is so big as to have a significant influence on the market price (consider beauty salons; most cities have a large number of them and no one salon or individual customer can exert control over the price or quantity of beauty treatments produced); (2) no collusion among the buyers or sellers to fix prices or quantities; (3) relatively free and easy entry into the market by new buyers or sellers; (4) no governmentally imposed restraints on prices or quantities; and (5) reasonably good information about price and quality known to buyers and sellers. Rather than rehash the arguments over whether these conditions apply to health care,[3] it is assumed that the trend of most public and private policies will continue to be aimed at correcting imperfections so that competition can more fully develop in the years ahead. Some additional barriers, however, will need to be overcome before the health care market can become truly competitive. Once these are discussed, issues pertaining to quality and nursing practice in a competitive environment can be more adequately examined.

PROBLEMS ON THE DEMAND SIDE
OF THE HEALTH CARE MARKET

Even when the aforementioned conditions for competition have been satisfied, its development among firms that supply health care services—health maintenance organizations (HMOs), preferred provider organizations (PPOs), prepaid health care plans, hospitals—will be hampered if buyers of health care are not sensitive to prices. Responding to an essay by Jones (1990), who argued that competition has been tried for 10 years through multiple choice health care plans without constraining costs, Enthoven (1990), a long-time advocate of competition in health care, wrote, "The plain fact is that employers have not tried 'competition' in the appropriate sense of the word" (p. 368). He provides the following explanation (pp. 368-369):

> Unfortunately, the word "competition" has led to much misunderstanding. Noneconomists understand "competition" to be present if there are multiple suppliers in a marketplace. Thus, one occasionally reads articles characterizing a market for hospital services as "very competitive" if there are many hospitals, without any reference to conditions on the demand side. When economists use the term, not modified by some other term such as "nonprice" or "service," they mean "price competition." Price competition is present only if alternative suppliers are offering their goods or services to purchasers who really care about price because they are using their own money and must give up something else of value if they choose to pay a higher price. In other words, for there to be price competition, the purchasers must be seeking value for their money. When we speak of market forces, free markets, and "the invisible hand," we are referring to economic systems in which there is price competition.

Indeed, much of the health care system has been built largely on what Enthoven (1988) terms "cost-unconscious" demand. The lack of sensitivity to the price of health care has occurred for several reasons, but perhaps the most important is the tax treatment of employer-paid health insurance premiums. Current tax law permits the exclusion of employer-paid health insurance premiums from employees' taxable income. This means that an employer can buy a greater amount of insurance (more benefits and more extensive coverage for a greater number of insurable events) for an employee than if the employee were given the same amount of money as wages, paid taxes on it, and then used what was left over to purchase health insurance. Consequently, this tax policy has resulted in the purchase of more health insurance coverage than would be the case if employees bought the insurance directly using after-tax income.[4] Furthermore, once an individual has health care insurance, the price of consuming health care services is minimal (although this is changing). This has resulted in an overconsumption (an inefficient demand) of medical care because employees are not conscious of the full price of the services they consume, and providers, who know that an insurance company, rather than the patient, will pay for the services, have had no economic incentive to restrain either the cost of providing a treatment or the amount of care provided. As long as the patient and provider are not sensitive to price and are spared from being fiscally responsible for their actions, patients will rationally demand more health care and providers will gladly supply it. Neither party has economic incentives to consider the costs or benefits of consuming additional amounts of medical care and behave as if more is better.

A second way that employers have fostered "cost-unconsciousness" is that, to date, most employers have constructed their health insurance offerings so that an employee who chooses the lowest-priced health plan is not permitted to keep any of the savings (Enthoven, 1990). Furthermore, "most employers systematically subsidize the more costly open-ended, fee-for-service third-party payer system against cost effective HMOs, thus attenuating or destroying the incentive for consumers to choose the more economical plan" (p. 370). This stymies price competition among health care plans (the suppliers) because lower-cost plans cannot "take business away from the next-lowest priced plan by cutting the price paid to the people actually making the choice" (p. 369). Enthoven and others (Brown, 1988; Iglehart, 1988) believe that employers persist with this irrational strategy because, in addition to the perverse incentives to purchase open-ended, fee-for-service plans inherent in the tax treatment of employer-paid health insurance premiums, unions have long insisted that their members have 100% employer-paid and comprehensive health coverage.[5] Further, because many employers perceive that the cost in terms of upsetting employees by insisting on cost-conscious choice in purchasing health care plans may not be worth the short-term savings, employers traditionally have been reluctant to use their considerable purchasing power to stimulate price competition among health care plans.

Demand Reforms

Although the number of HMOs and competitive health care plans is expected to grow, as well as the percentage of the population enrolled, these plans will not become price competitive and achieve the desired cost-minimizing performance until they are driven by the need to satisfy cost-conscious purchasers. For this to happen, changes on the demand side of the market are necessary.[6] To McClure (Iglehart, 1988, pp. 80-81) these changes mean implementing a "Buy Right" strategy, which he describes as:

> getting the patients and purchasers (employers, union trust funds, Medicare, and so forth) to buy in the right way: very specific ways that force the providers and plans to compete on quality, humaneness, and efficiency. . . . This strategy is based on the notion that if you want providers and plans to compete on quality and efficiency, then you have to reward those who have it and punish those who don't. The only way to reward a provider or plan for efficiency and quality is with more patients. This is also the right way to reward them because it propagates good performance throughout the system.

To achieve demand reform, large purchasers, such as unions and employers, and even individual consumers must have economic incentives to consider the cost of these plans. These incentives could take the form of allowing purchasers to keep any savings accrued from making economical choices, requiring deductibles, copayments, or both, limiting employees to the use of only nontaxed, excluded income, or capping the amount of excluded income they may use to purchase health care insurance. Demand reform also will require employers and unions to become much better informed about what they are buying and begin to manage purchases of health care plans as if they were any other business expense. In addition to economic incentives that take into account the cost of health care plans, purchasers also must have information on the quality of each plan. Knowing each plan's price and having information on its quality will enable purchasers to make more informed buying decisions; it is the only way to pressure the plans to minimize costs while simultaneously and constantly seeking ways to improve quality. To illustrate, consider an HMO competing against other HMOs or prepaid health plans. Because the HMO must keep its costs low to retain a portion of the prepaid amount, it will contract with the least costly hospital(s) to provide care for plan members whenever indicated. This puts pressure on hospitals to be cost minimizers so they can be awarded contracts with competing health plans and thereby obtain access to patient populations and keep their beds filled. The HMO, however, will not enter into an arrangement with a hospital solely on the basis of low cost, but will consider the hospital's reputation and indicators of the quality of care it provides. The HMO is concerned with quality because it risks losing members if they are dissatisfied with hospital care (or any other provider used by the HMO). Because members of the HMO can quit the plan and join a competitor with a better reputation, the HMO cannot afford to skimp on quality simply to lower its costs.[7] In this way cost-minimizing and quality-improving behaviors are transmitted throughout the system.

Beyond the problems associated with the lack of the purchaser's sensitivity to the cost of health care plans, perverse incentives contained in the tax treatment of employer-paid health insurance, union pressures for comprehensive coverage, and employer hesitancy to become more aggressive in purchasing health care plans on the basis of cost and quality, there are other problems affecting efficiency on the demand side of the market. Some of these problems concern overcoming adverse or bias risk selection (to minimize costs, plans would prefer to enroll younger and relatively healthy people, leaving older or sicker people for other health plans to insure); standardizing a base or common benefits package (which would make comparisons between plans feasible); determining how best to include the uninsured in a system of competing health care plans; and deciding on the proper roles for government and employers in promoting and managing competition among plans (Enthoven & Kronick, 1989). It is beyond the scope of this chapter, however, to discuss these problems or to examine the options that have been proposed to overcome them. Suffice it to say that a substantial amount of large-scale research is being done on these problems (unfortunately, very little by nurses) and little consensus has emerged thus far on how they will be resolved.[8] On the other hand, as employers continue to experience increasing health care costs and to bear the consequent effect on undermining the ability to be price competitive in an increasingly global marketplace, it is reasonable to anticipate that they will become more motivated to achieve demand reforms and support greater competition among health care plans. It is in the best interests of the nursing profession, therefore, to become much more involved in research and management efforts that seek to find solutions to these problems.

COMPETITION AND THE QUALITY OF HEALTH CARE

Because people are concerned that quality will deteriorate in a price competitive system, Feldstein (1988b) contends that both providers and purchasers will be especially cautious and willing to take steps to ensure high quality. Thus, if anything, quality is likely to improve as a result of increased competition. Recalling that firms in a competitive market must provide goods and services that satisfy consumers' preferences and perceptions of quality, it is not surprising that, even with the limited extent to which price competition has heretofore developed in health care, today there is intense research interest and management activity in quality of care. (This is quite different from the past when health care providers and professionals controlled information about quality and created an impression, perhaps even a misleading impression, of high quality health care.) Furthermore, it is no coincidence that contemporary writers (Caper, 1988; Davies & Ware, 1988; Ellwood & Paul, 1986; Francis, 1986; Lohr, Yordy, & Thier, 1988) uniformly stress the importance of incorporating indicators of consumers' satisfaction and not just professional determination of quality in the development and testing of quality assessment tools. Perhaps it is for these reasons that Ellwood and Paul (1986) wrote, "Competition, maligned by some as narrow-visioned cost cutting and a threat to quality, is now driving the movement toward genuine quality management" (p. 138). Indeed, competition in health care is neither logically inconsistent nor incompatible with high quality health services; competition does, however, pose a threat to firms and professionals who do not provide high quality care.

IMPLICATIONS FOR NURSING

As competition develops more fully in health care, it is reasonable to anticipate that providers and purchasers will behave increasingly like the model described in the beginning of this chapter. Health care providers will have strong economic incentives to be innovative in their use of resources in order to minimize production costs and price their products competitively, will constantly be attempting to improve the quality of products and services, will conduct extensive market research, and will undertake promotional initiatives to inform purchasers on the price and quality of their health care products. If substantial demand reform occurs, purchasers of health care will be better informed about the quality of health care plans and will have economic incentives to shop around for the least costly plan for a given level of quality. On the basis of this scenario of market competition in health care, in the years ahead nursing can anticipate the following implications:

1. Intensifying pressures to provide nursing care in the least costly manner
2. Increasing demand by licensed practical nurses (LPNs), clinical pharmacists, physicians, and other economic competitors for regulations that either protect or expand their practice "turfs," coupled with actions by employers to change state nursing practice acts and institutional traditions that restrict them from achieving productivity gains and lowering labor-related costs
3. Developing opportunities to advance the value of nursing practice in all health care settings if the profession's research and management communities can successfully orchestrate a multifaceted quality assessment effort
4. Struggling to balance the tensions, costs, and benefits between

pursuing a narrowly focused nursing quality assessment strategy
and finding ways to integrate nursing quality assessment concepts
and methods into already existing and developing quality assessment systems and management initiatives that are controlled
largely by persons who are not nurses

5. Having to seriously consider what it is that purchasers and consumers want from nursing and taking steps to satisfy these wants

The remainder of this chapter discusses some of the challenges and
opportunities arising from these implications.

Pressures to Reduce Costs

Concurrent with the system becoming more competitive, health care
providers will attempt to gain a thorough understanding of the costs of
producing their products and services. Providers who do not have good
information on their production costs, or whose costs are high, will
jeopardize their ability to be price competitive. Nursing therefore can
anticipate that provider-employers will have mounting financial incentives to do whatever is required to better understand their cost structure
and to take appropriate actions to minimize costs.

Cost-reducing strategies will vary by type of health care provider, by
extent to which inefficiencies exist, by availability of opportunities to
realize economies of scale, and by degree to which price competition
governs market conditions and management behavior. For some firms,
reducing costs will be accomplished best by taking advantage of economies of scale, which could mean that a firm will down-size (which could
lead to loss of employment for nurses), whereas for others lower costs
may be achieved by becoming larger, perhaps by merging with or joining
a chain of similar firms (which could lead to increased employment
opportunities for nurses). In large urban areas in which market competition is likely to be more prevalent and well developed, pressures to
reduce costs are likely to be greater than in rural or other areas in which
competition is less developed. More directly important to nurses, however, will be the actions of large employers that specifically focus on
minimizing labor-related costs and eliminating inefficiencies. For example, should hospital management insist on proof that employing more
highly educated nurses, namely those with baccalaureate nursing degrees, helps lower costs, how will nursing service administrators respond? Empirical evidence supporting this relationship is lacking, and it
is also unclear that the employment of nursing staffs consisting only of
registered nurses (RNs) is efficient or makes strong economic sense. As
providers' economic survival becomes directly tied to their ability to
lower costs (so they can price their services competitively), nursing administrators can expect either to demonstrate the cost effectiveness of
employing more highly educated nurses or possibly to contend with

hospital managers who take matters into their own hands, some of whom may be guided by the notion that "a nurse is a nurse is a nurse." These employers may even conclude that the only way to reduce labor-related nursing costs is to begin programs that train RN substitutes to provide essentially the same nursing care but at lower cost. The American Medical Association's attempt to develop registered care technologists (RCTs) and the American Hospital Association's support of training programs to develop multi-skilled health practitioners demonstrate that responses of this kind are not without precedent.

Rather than gamble that managers will take such actions, nurse administrators may wish to view mounting cost pressures as an opportunity to gain management's support and involvement to undertake a critical self-appraisal of current nursing practice patterns and organizational arrangements. An objective and comprehensive examination is likely to reveal any number of tasks, clinical procedures, and unit policies that only marginally contribute to patient care, that are outdated and cost ineffective, and that are dissatisfying to nurses and patients.[9] Working with hospital management to eliminate these holdovers of nursing care may result in substantial cost savings, improve the quality of patient care, and increase management's understanding of the issues, problems, and rewards associated with nursing. In addition, those conducting research in nursing service administration have an opportunity to make much needed contributions by reconceiving and implementing nursing unit management structures and working closely with clinicians to determine their cost effectiveness and impact on nurses and achievement of patient outcomes.

Pressures to Change Regulations Governing Nursing Practice

To avoid the political and economic costs associated with the aforementioned plan to develop RN-substitute staffs, large employers of nurses may attempt to change either state practice acts or institutional traditions that prevent them from employing the least costly mix of nurse and nonnurse human resources. Indeed, Feldstein (1988a) has documented the many ways that legal restrictions governing the practice of health care professionals have resulted in fewer providers, higher prices, and less innovation in the delivery of health care services (for examples, see footnote 3). Thus, just as nurse practitioners, nurse anesthetists, and nurse-midwives have sought changes in state practice acts to advance their economic and practice interests, employers can be expected to seek changes in legal restrictions governing the tasks that can be performed by other health care personnel if they believe that present restrictions result in higher labor costs. Examples of areas in which employers may seek regulatory changes include the removal of restrictions requiring that an RN must always be on duty, maintenance of certain RN to LPN staffing ratios, and preventing LPNs (and even nurse aides) from administering medications or performing procedures currently done by RNs. The nursing profession can anticipate that LPNs, pharmacy technicians, and others who stand to gain from lifting these types of restrictions will join with employers to exert political pressure on state regulatory agencies and legislators to make the desired changes.[10] If RNs attempt to counter these political actions by recycling traditional arguments that justify regulations on the premise that they are needed to ensure high-quality health care and protect the public, they are likely to find them far less effective in a health care environment governed by price competition. Furthermore, if developing methods of quality assessment focus more on outcomes of care and less on the process of care, as current trends indicate, then regulations governing the inputs or process of providing nursing care, such as those already noted, may be challenged for the very reason that there is no evidence linking them to attaining desired quality of care outcomes! Thus, in a price competitive market in which providers bear the full cost of their decisions, nursing can anticipate that employers will be increasingly willing to allocate the time, energy, and resources to seek changes in state regulations and institutional restrictions governing nursing practice if they believe that this will help minimize costs without sacrificing quality.

Increasing the Profession's Value Through Quality Assessment of Nursing Care

The opportunity presented by pressures to reduce costs and to eliminate restrictions placed on RN competitors is, of course, for the profession to demonstrate its cost effectiveness, enhance nurse managers' performance and control over resources consumed by nursing units, and provide desired patient outcomes. For this to happen, however, a vigorous and intertwined research and management effort in two areas should ensue. The first involves evaluating the efficiency of various organizational innovations for delivering nursing care in both acute and nonacute health care systems. Fortunately, a good part of this work is now under way through the innovations being developed and evaluated in the 20 inpatient and community demonstration sites jointly funded by the Robert Wood Johnson Foundation and Pew Memorial Trust program to strengthen nursing care, as well as by related projects funded by the National Center for Nursing Research. It will be important for nursing administrators and educators to promote the diffusion of innovations that result from these initiatives.

The second area of needed research and management effort involves empirically demonstrating the cost effectiveness of nursing interventions. Success in this area requires a definition of nursing interventions and expected outcomes that, to the extent possible, explicitly reflect nursing's unique focus on the whole individual (versus parts or diseases) and its clinical activities that assist patients' responses to illness. The work of

McCloskey et al. (1990) is well under way in developing a classification of nursing interventions, but studies that demonstrate significant clinical outcomes and financial savings that result from well-designed nursing interventions are critically needed. Research and management effort in these two key areas will explicate the profession's clinical and economic value.

One of the benefits of undertaking effort in these areas is that the nursing profession will have a much better understanding of its cost structure both at a unit level and at the level of specific clinical interventions. This will give nursing administrators the knowledge needed to make cost-effective management decisions, which, in turn, should help minimize the potential threats posed by employers and RN competitors discussed earlier. In addition, by validating outcomes and understanding their costs, the profession will position itself to be considered more favorably not only by hospital management but by HMOs, competitive health plans, large employers, and insurers. It is a mistake to assume that health care plan managers and financiers have more than a superficial understanding of nursing. If they can be educated about nursing's philosophy of viewing people as whole beings and understand the basis of its clinical interventions, it is conceivable that plan managers may see nursing care as representing an "innovation" that is clinically more appropriate and less costly for managing a substantial portion of their enrollees' health care needs. Thus, to the extent that nursing has unambiguously defined its interventions and outcomes (in terms that the public and purchasers understand) and has developed reliable and valid methods to assess them, the value of the profession's "stock" could increase substantially. Skeptics of this potential should keep in mind that as health care plans and other providers begin to compete on price and become increasingly motivated to reduce costs without jeopardizing quality, they will have strong financial incentives to seriously consider a well-conceived nursing strategy. Also, if skeptics believe that physicians will succeed in preventing nursing from gaining more than a foothold in competitive health care plans, then they do not realize that these plans can be expected to exert an opposite, if not overwhelming, political force to see that the payer has access to lower-cost innovations, regardless of whose professional ox is gored. After all, if the payer does not recognize innovations that lower costs, competing health care plans risk going out of business.

Integrating Nursing Quality Care Assessment With the Work of Non-Nurses

As substantial and appealing as are the potential benefits of pursuing a research and management effort aimed at effecting the quality and establishing the cost effectiveness of nursing care, nurses engaged in this work must be cognizant that neither quality assessment nor the science of evaluation that underlies this activity belongs to nursing and that quality assessment of health care is a much larger social good whose attainment can come about only when the contributions of all health care professions are understood and appropriately integrated. If unique, stand-alone (and costly) quality of care assessment methods, computer software programs, and related data bases are developed for the sole benefit of nurses, then the profession may not be able to easily integrate its quality assessment concepts and technology into other assessment systems that are being developed by insurers, hospitals, physicians, and competitive health care plans. Should nursing choose neither to work with non-nurses nor to participate in mutually evaluating the outcomes of nursing and medical care, it risks being excluded from ongoing and future research and demonstration programs or, if included in them, being relegated to filling only minor roles. Thus leaders of nursing quality assessment research and management efforts must find ways to become part of medically oriented quality assessment initiatives. This can be accomplished by working with physicians and making better use of health insurance claims data and other large data bases. Working with non-nurses is an excellent way to educate them about the special and not so special aspects of nursing, and it also is an important way for nurses to learn from others.

A final argument for working with other health professions in assessing the quality of nursing care is that in the future there are likely to be private and federal actions to adopt uniform quality assessment systems either on a regional basis or nationwide. A uniform quality assessment system would save time and money, permit meaningful comparisons of quality data, and enable longitudinal evaluations of the outcomes of care (Ellwood, 1988). Nursing therefore cannot afford to pursue its quality of care assessment effort in isolation lest it risk being inadequately represented in evolving uniform assessment systems. Neither can nursing afford to surrender the opportunity to discover the scientific basis of its unique perspective and validate its clinical interventions by subsuming to a larger, medically oriented quality assessment system. Somehow the profession must pursue its quality assessment agenda so that it is narrow enough to preserve and strengthen the uniqueness of nursing, yet broad enough to be applicable and comfortably situated within a rapidly evolving and comprehensive quality of care assessment system.

Understanding What Consumers Want From Nursing

An overriding theme of this chapter's discussion of market competition is that firms compete not only on the basis of price but also on the strength of their reputations and the quality of their goods and services. It has been argued that in the future, purchasers of personal health care services and of health insurance plans will demand much more information about quality than they do today and that perceptions of quality will play an increasingly important role in their choices. This will reinforce competition among health care plans and providers. It also is likely that providers who attain a reputation for high quality will be able to enlarge their share of the market and may even be able to charge higher prices because some purchasers are willing to pay a little more for what they perceive as higher quality.[11]

Given the emerging importance of quality, it is important for the nursing profession to recognize that it can obtain a strategic advantage over other health professionals if it begins to make a concerted and systematic effort to better understand what quality nursing care means to purchasers and what they want from nurses. In this sense, purchasers of nursing services would include insurance companies, employers, unions, and individual consumers. Understanding what it is about nursing that satisfies purchasers not only will enable nurses to develop closer relationships with them but also will guide nurses in making structural and clinical changes to better provide the type of nursing care purchasers find most satisfying. Stated in businesslike terms, nurses concerned with the provision of clinical care should undertake market research to clarify who, in fact, is its market (as well as who is likely to be its market in the future), as well as what the market wants and how nurses should go about providing it. To survive in a competitive marketplace, suppliers of health care (nurses in independent practice or hospitals that employ RNs) must offer services that satisfy purchasers. Satisfaction means that purchasers will be willing to give up something of value in exchange for nursing care that combines an optimal mix of humanistic and technical activities with well-defined and measurable outcomes.

Finally, in collecting quality of care data, it is important to avoid using only nursing's professional definitions of quality. Rather, assessment tools should encourage consumers and give them ways to indicate the interpersonal dimensions of quality that they find satisfying and dissatisfying. Davies and Ware (1988) provide an excellent discussion of the arguments for and against using consumer data in assessing quality of care, and they conclude that "indeed, data from consumers undoubtedly represent the centerpiece of any effort to examine the interpersonal component of quality. Regarding the technical process of care, reports and ratings from consumers likely will provide a valuable supplement to data from more traditional sources such as the medical record" (p. 45). A word of caution: although incorporating the patient's point of view in defining and measuring quality health care is indeed a positive development and is consistent with a market orientation to health care, if taken to its extreme there could be drawbacks. For example, concerned that highly satisfied patients may be induced to stay with health care plans, Brook and Kosecoff (1988) warn that as competition intensifies, "money and effort that might have been spent on improving quality will be spent on improving satisfaction regardless of whether or not this translates into future improvements in patient health status" (p. 155).

CONCLUSION

Competition rewards those who bring to the marketplace goods and services that are priced "right" and that satisfy purchasers' demands. By recognizing the economic incentives underlying an emerging price-competitive health care marketplace, taking steps to make nursing cost effective, and conducting a well-conceived quality of care assessment effort, nurses can target the purchasers of health care now, while they are coming out of their relatively cost "unconscious" state, and bring forth new management ideas and clinical strategies that will advance the profession in the years ahead. The future health care environment can be more receptive to nursing and more rewarding if its quality assessment leaders work closely with nurse administrators to help the profession become more responsive to the needs of those who purchase nursing services. Competition, unlike the former regulatory strategy that governed much of the economic activity in health care in the past, will handsomely reward those who innovate and take risks.

FOOTNOTES

1. In 1982 the Supreme Court upheld a 1978 lower court decision that ruled in favor of the Federal Trade Commission's 1975 charge that the American Medical Association and its constituent medical societies had engaged in anticompetitive behavior. Feldstein (1988a) writes that the Supreme Court's decision "was a clear signal to health professions that they would now be subject to the antitrust laws" (p. 313), thereby legitimizing competition in health care. The socially desirable outcomes of competition include greater incentives for hospital efficiency, less duplication of costly facilities and services, minimizing the cost of a medical treatment, increased physician productivity, greater incentives for more preventive care and health education, greater use of generic drugs, and innovations in the delivery of medical care. (See Feldstein [1988a, Chapter 12] for a more comprehensive description of the benefits and expected outcomes of competition in medical care.)
2. Clearly, for some goods that are relatively inexpensive and do not affect a buyer's overall budget to a significant degree (paper clips, laundry detergent, motor oil), consumers usually are willing to pay a few cents more for the product rather than to incur the costs associated with traveling and spending time searching for the lowest price. On the other hand, if the good is stereo equipment or a television set, which are more expensive and if purchased would represent a greater impact on the consumer's budget, then consumers have an economic incentive to search for the lowest price.
3. It is important to note, however, that a regulatory strategy has been successfully used by health professionals and providers to keep these conditions from developing and thereby prevent price competition. For example, hospitals used Certificate of Need (CoN) regulations to restrict the growth in the number of other "sellers" (hospitals, especially proprietary hospitals, HMOs, and ambulatory surgery centers). Rather than take direct action to collude among themselves, hospitals manipulated the CoN process

to retard rival hospitals from obtaining new technology and, with respect to nursing, Yett (1975) reports that in the past hospitals have colluded to fix nurse wages through wage stabilization programs. In addition, hospitals have exerted political pressure on regulatory agencies to erect barriers to prevent new providers (e.g., HMOs, hospices, and surgicenters) from entering the market. Physicians and dentists have obtained legal restrictions by means of state practice acts to prevent nurse practitioners, nurse-midwives, physician assistants, optometrists, chiropractors, denturists, dental hygienists and assistants, and others from entering "their" markets. State insurance boards have not allowed nurse practitioners to receive direct payment for their services—which would have enabled them to compete directly with physicians, increase the overall amount of health care available to the public, and give the public a greater number of choices in the health care professionals from which it could select to receive personal health care services. Further, physicians and dentists have fostered "ethical restrictions" and used state practice acts to prevent practitioners from advertising the price and quality of services, although such restrictions have been ruled anticompetitive and illegal by the courts.

4. The secretary of the Department of Health and Human Services reported that the cost of this tax exclusion is $58 billion annually (*Medicine and Health*, 1990). This amount represents a tremendous cost to the federal government in terms of forgone tax revenue. As the federal government seeks ways to reduce the budget, the modification of this tax exclusion will become increasingly possible so that all or part of these revenues can flow to the government and not to health insurers. One can anticipate, however, that unions, upper middle–class employees, and insurers will mount considerable effort to keep the exclusion, as would health care providers who likely would suffer a decreased demand for their services if the exclusion were removed. For a more complete discussion of this tax policy and its implications on efficiency and equity, see Feldstein (1988a) or Brown (1988).

5. A recent study by the Health Insurance Association found that 77% of companies with more than 100 employees continue to offer among their coverage options traditional indemnity, or fee-for-service health plans, which have proved resistant to most cost-control efforts. The study reports that about 70% of employees in the United States are covered under traditional plans, with the remainder enrolled in HMOs and PPOs, although these percentages may have increased since the study was completed.

6. Although not all the problems on the supply side of the health care market are resolved, McClure (Iglehart, 1988) asserts that supply reform—the integration of providers and insurers into competing comprehensive health care plans, such as HMOs, PPOs, independent practice associations (IPAs), and managed insurance plans—is well under way and will continue to grow. In addition, competition on the supply side will be enhanced by significant excess capacity among hospitals, reflected by occupancy rates averaging less than 70%. The growing supply of physicians is contributing to an increase of excess capacity, which also will promote more competitive behavior. Assuming no perverse payment methods exist that would provide payment of the costs associated with unfilled hospital beds, hospitals with excess capacity would have strong economic incentives to fill their empty beds by engaging in competitive actions designed to attract patients away from other hospitals. Similarly, physicians would be more likely to compete with other physicians to increase the number of patient visits.

7. Francis (1986) sought to determine the effects of cost competition and service quality on HMO growth (e.g., service quality reflects clients' satisfaction with waiting time for appointments, ability to select a health professional of one's choice, satisfaction with the professional and personal skills of the professional used, convenience of hours, perceived appropriateness of treatment). Multiple regression analysis was used to examine the effects of predictor variables on the quit rate per 100 persons reported by HMOs participating in the Federal Employee Health Benefits Program. With use of data

on 151 health care plans and on the basis of seven predictor variables in the regression equation, an R-square of .15 was obtained, which was statistically significant at the .0001 level. The most important predictor variable was the expected costs to enrollees. Because variables measuring service satisfaction were unavailable and thus not used in the regression analysis, Francis concluded, "It appears that the great majority of the unexplained difference (in quit rates for each plan) represents service dimensions." These results support the view that plan enrollees will vote with their feet if the HMO becomes too costly (they will switch to lower cost plans) or if they are dissatisfied with service (quality) features.

8. Major research projects on quality of care are described by Heinen, Gorski, and Roe (1988), none of which included a nurse as a principal or coinvestigator, or a nursing organization as the recipient of funding or other type of involvement.

9. A recent study (Buerhaus, 1991) of Michigan RNs found that, regardless of education, full- or part-time employment status, or employment setting, RNs believed that task requirements of the job and organizational policies were the least important components of work satisfaction. In addition, with the exception of pay, RNs were least satisfied with these two components. Sovie (1989) identifies a useful list of what she calls "nursing's sacred cows" and provides an excellent discussion of how to "slaughter" dissatisfying and useless task requirements and organizational policies.

10. Another regulatory implication concerns nurse practitioners and changes affecting physicians. The steadily increasing supply of physicians and strong payment reform measures enacted by Congress pose significant threats to nurses with advanced degrees who are attempting to practice more autonomously. This will come about because, as the number of physicians grows, they will not be able to use all of their available time and resources to their fullest and most productive potential. To increase their productivity and make full use of capacity (and thereby increase or at least maintain their incomes), physicians will find that they must increasingly compete on the basis of price and on the ability to provide medical care that satisfies consumers' wants and preferences. Advertising will flourish, especially by younger physicians who are at a competitive disadvantage and who may be less willing to go along with the medical profession's traditional "ethical guidelines" deploring its use. Fueling this competition will be the tightening vise of federal policies that will constrain the amount of federal spending available to a growing number of physicians and further threaten their incomes. Nurse practitioners, midwives, and others intent on independent practice can expect that they will have to do more market research and advertising to compete for patients and that regulatory or legislative efforts to require direct payment for services (or attempts to take it away in areas in which this is already occurring) will be firmly resisted by physicians, because such a policy would add to the number of competitors and further erode their incomes.

11. This has already occurred in health care as demonstrated by teaching hospitals that have successfully used their reputation for providing high-quality health care to defend a higher cost structure and to obtain higher payments than do nonteaching hospitals.

REFERENCES

Boyar, D. C. (1985). Will a healthy dose of competition cure the health-care system's ills? *Nursing Economics, 3*, 234-237.

Brook, R. H., & Kosecoff, J. B. (1988). Competition and quality. *Health Affairs, 7*(3), 133-149.

Brown, L. D. (1988). *Health policy in the United States: Issues and options.* (Occasional Paper 4, Ford Foundation Project on Social Welfare and the American Future). New York: Ford Foundation.

Buerhaus, P. I. (in press). Linking the economic and nursing perspectives on shortage of registered nurses. *Journal of Health Politics, Policy, and Law.*

Caper, P. (1988). Defining quality in medical care. *Health Affairs*, 7(1), 49-61.

Davies, A. R., & Ware, J. E. (1988). Involving consumers in quality assessment. *Health Affairs*, 7(1), 33-48.

Ellwood, P. M., & Paul, B. A. (1986). But what about quality? *Health Affairs*, 5(1), 135-140.

Ellwood, P. M. (1988). Special report. Shattuck Lecture—Outcomes management. A technology of patient experience. *New England Journal of Medicine, 318*, 1549-1556.

Enthoven, A. C. (1988). Managed competition: An agenda for action. *Health Affairs*, 7(3), 25-47.

Enthoven, A. C. (1990). Multiple choice health insurance: The lessons and challenges to employers. *Inquiry, 27*, 368-373.

Enthoven, A. C., & Kronick, R. (1989). A consumer choice health plan for the 1990s: Universal health insurance in a system designed to promote quality and economy. *New England Journal of Medicine, 320*, 29-37; 94-101.

Feldstein, P. (1988a). *Health care economics* (3rd ed.). Albany, NY: Delmar.

Feldstein, P. (1988b). *The politics of health legislation: An economic perspective*. Ann Arbor, MI: Health Administration Press Perspectives.

Francis, W. (1986). HMO customer service. *Health Affairs*, 5(1), 173-182.

Fuchs, V. R. (1988). The "competition revolution" in health care. *Health Affairs*, 7(3), 5-24.

Havighurst, C. C. (1983). The doctors' trust: Self-regulation and the law. *Health Affairs*, 2(3), 64-76.

Heinen, L. A., Gorski, J. A., & Roe, W. (1988). Quality of care research and projects in progress. *Health Affairs*, 7(1), 145-150.

Iglehart, J. K. (1988). Competition and the pursuit of quality: A conversation with Walter McClure. *Health Affairs*, 7(1), 79-90.

Jones, S. B. (1990). Multiple choice health insurance: The lessons and challenge to private insurers. *Inquiry, 27*(2), 161-166.

Lohr, K. N., Yordy, K. D., & Thier, S. (1988). Current issues in quality of care. *Health Affairs*, 7(1), 5-18.

McCloskey, J. C., Bulecheck, G. M., Cohen, M. Z., Craft, M. J., Crossley, J. D., Denehy, J. A., Glick, O. J., Kruckeberg, T., Maas, M., Prophet, C. M., & Tripp-Reimer, T. (1990). Classification of nursing interventions. *Journal of Professional Nursing, 6*(3), 151-157.

Relman, A. (1983). The future of medical practice. *Health Affairs*, 2(2), 5-19.

Sovie, M. D. (1989). Clinical nursing practices and patient outcomes: Evaluation, evolution, and revolution (Legitimizing radical change to maximize nurses' time for quality care). *Nursing Economics*, 7(2), 79-85.

Yett, D. (1975). *An economic analysis of the nursing shortage*. Toronto, ON: D. C. Heath.

CHAPTER 3

Collaboration for Quality:
The Next Step in Health Care

Patricia Schroeder

Interdisciplinary collaboration is essential for effective quality assurance initiatives. Although accountability for many patient outcomes is shared among disciplines, quality assurance programs traditionally have been carried out within individual disciplines or departments. Factors necessary for collaboration efforts suggest the need for radical changes in many health care organizations and for philosophic changes among professionals.

THE VALUE OF INTERDISCIPLINARY COLLABORATION

Collaboration among disciplines in the health care setting greatly affects the achievement of positive patient outcomes. An often-quoted study from George Washington University School of Medicine addressed the care of patients in intensive care units at 13 tertiary care hospitals. After extensive data collection on patient, therapeutic, and organizational variables, it was identified that one of the significant factors determining positive outcomes was interaction and communication between physicians and nurses (Knaus, Draper, Wagner, & Zimmerman, 1986). This study substantiated what practicing nurses have already known—that

Quality Care Concepts Inc., 524 BelAire Drive, Thiensville, WI 53092.

Series on Nursing Administration—Volume III, 1992

quality health care can be achieved only through a coordinated effort by professionals. Although the contributions of each professional discipline must be provided safely, effectively, and efficiently, an additional step must be taken to coordinate care into an organized and integrated whole. The impact of what can be achieved collaboratively is much greater than simply the sum of the individual efforts. Interdisciplinary collaboration is essential for quality care.

Interdisciplinary collaboration also is essential for effective quality assurance (QA) programs. To date, however, quality-related programs that are truly collaborative are rare. We have moved forward in our ability to define, measure, and improve the quality of care in terms of individual disciplines. This has been and will continue to be a necessary achievement. We have failed, however, to simultaneously move forward in creating programs and relationships to support collaboration for quality. Often, hospital-wide QA committees function as a clearinghouse for departmental reports rather than as a forum for synthesis, leadership, and strategic planning for quality. Efforts have focused on timeliness, volume of reports, and meeting the minimum expectations of the Joint Commission on Accreditation of Healthcare Organizations (Joint Commission) rather than on creating an organizational culture that supports and expects professionals to work together in improving care.

The pursuit of clinical quality in traditional QA programs has been carried out almost solely within individual disciplines or departments. Professionals commonly address quality issues that reflect their most significant contributions to care, as they see them. Actions taken to improve care typically remain within the domain of the discipline. Tunnel vision has resulted, narrowing perspective and stifling creativity and potential. Some clinical departments are mandated by the Joint Commission to demonstrate multidisciplinary QA activities (special care units such as intensive care, burn units, renal dialysis units, neonatal intensive care). Yet it is not unusual to hear of problems ranging from limited success to completely ineffective programs.

Often accountability for many necessary patient outcomes is shared among disciplines. To monitor and evaluate these outcomes without an atmosphere or a program structure supportive of interdisciplinary collaboration is inefficient at best and destructive at worst. As health care becomes more focused on outcome, the creation of QA programs with the expectation of and support for collaboration becomes increasingly necessary.

REASONS FOR UNILATERAL QUALITY ASSURANCE FOCUS

Although the value of collaboration is significant, there have been many reasons why QA programs with a unilateral focus have evolved. Nurses have been more involved in quality assurance than professionals in other disciplines, creating programs and activities that have been in place longer and have included more staff members than many other departments. Nurses often have a better understanding of the QA process than do other health care professionals. As employees of organizations that have regulatory and accrediting expectations, nurses have felt the obligation to participate in QA programs, thus being pushed beyond their own professional and personal accountability. Finally, and unfortunately, too many QA programs have been established solely to meet Joint Commission expectations, or to look good on paper, or to carry out a bureaucratic function rather than to improve care or practice. When multidisciplinary groups are established for these reasons, true collaboration is not achieved and the groups rarely make an impact on quality issues.

There have been too many missed opportunities within our unilateral QA programs. We have missed the potential for solving some significant clinical problems because of political agendas, present in part because of lack of positive relationships with other disciplines. We have missed the ability to communicate what we know to be the patient's perspective about quality care. We have lost a forum to articulate the unique and important role that nurses play in achieving positive outcomes of care. Although we have spent time attempting to differentiate one department's turf from another, we have missed the point of QA—improving care for patients.

Imagine the potential of a nursing QA activity targeted to address problems with patient preparation and education for discharge. Certainly, the nursing department alone could undertake changes that would improve patient outcomes. Yet greater improvements could result, if nurses ultimately could convince others (disciplines, departments, systems) to change their approaches. Now imagine the potential of collaborative efforts involving all appropriate disciplines and departments as part of the initial efforts. The resulting ideas and efforts could be synergistic. If everyone were invested in the necessity of addressing this clinical issue, the impact could be much greater. Collaboration for quality could be highly effective.

To clarify, collaboration does not happen automatically by virtue of multidisciplinary group membership. Weiss and Davis (1985, p. 299) suggest that collaboration is the "interactions between nurse and physician that enable the knowledge and skills of both professionals to synergistically influence the patient care being provided," Kohles and Barry (1989, p. 9) differentiate joint responsibility from the collaborative process. They suggest that joint responsibility promotes unilateral functioning and one-way communication regarding two disciplines working on the same clinical issue. The collaborative process, instead, is "an interactive model of cooperation that allowed for exploration of the values brought by each discipline and a recognition of the importance of those values in problem identification and their influence on outcome expectations."

Precipitating collaboration, then, is not a simple or straightforward task. Collaboration for the improvement of quality of care is difficult.

Some of the most ardent attempts at multidisciplinary QA have failed because, in fact, they were not collaborative at all. These included such approaches as nurses collecting data about another discipline's practice, one discipline identifying the problems or suggesting strategies for changing another, and several disciplines evaluating the care of their colleagues as provided to the same patient population. Given the previous definitions of collaboration, these attempts have fallen far short.

FACTORS NECESSARY FOR COLLABORATION

Puta (1989) identifies factors necessary for collaboration. These include Devereux's suggestions (1981) of clinical competence, accountability, cooperativeness, assertiveness, receptivity to and respect for the other professional's contributions, and the ability to negotiate. Puta also notes organizational factors, which include nursing support systems, as well as the support of administrative and medical staff leadership.

The presence or creation of such factors suggests a radical shift in the culture of many health care organizations. This shift would require the creation of an enduring philosophy that values both quality and those who provide and receive care. It would require the creation of an enduring process that allows for and even demands the improvement of quality across disciplines and systems.

Evolution of the conduct of QA programs in health care has closely paralleled the expectations of the Joint Commission. Approximately every 5 years a major shift has occurred in the process of carrying out QA activities on the basis of the Joint Commission's standards. Recently, however, the philosophies of quality improvement espoused and used in other industries have created great interest because of their track record of success. Many health care organizations have begun implementing quality improvement programs based on the teachings of Deming (Crosby, 1979; Ishikawa, 1985; Juran, 1988; Peters, 1987; Walton, 1986). Even the Joint Commission's Agenda for Change has incorporated the philosophy of continuous improvement as part of its premise (Joint Commission, 1990).

QUALITY IMPROVEMENT

It is interesting to note that, in many practice settings currently implementing quality improvement (QI) programs as well as quality assurance (QA) programs, these programs are parallel and not integrated. That is, they are conducted independently by use of separate staff and separate resources, and they follow separate leadership and lines of reporting. One nurse described these programs by saying that quality assurance is necessary for accrediting purposes and quality improvement is intended to make a difference in practice and care. This is an unfortunate but common perception. Somehow we have lost the vision that quality assurance is meant to improve care. Because of the inadequacies of our conduct of traditional QA programs, we have felt the need to create new programs rather than enhance the philosophy and conduct of what is already present. The duplication and unnecessary use of resources that result in having one ineffective and one effective program are wasteful in today's fiscally constrained health care industry.

CONCLUSION

The ultimate goal for any quality-related program in health care today must be to empower those who practice within the setting to continuously improve care and service for patient well-being. To that end, we must look at how to create a collaborative approach to quality, without losing the autonomy and unique contributions of the professions. We cannot and should not stop our work in nursing QA programs but should instead build components of the program that support true collaboration. Health care organizations must establish a leadership commitment for quality and engage managers and staff (at all levels) in the ultimate importance of this pursuit. Education regarding quality and the processes for its measurement and achievement must be provided. Patient needs and outcomes must be a central focus, given the mission of the organization and the professional commitment of health care professionals.

In addition, we must learn to work together effectively in groups. Roles in groups should be clearly defined. Leaders and followers in groups must be treated as equals, with equal value and equally necessary roles to fulfill. Rewards of quality improvement must be equally shared.

As nurses we have come a long way in our capacity to define, measure, and improve the quality of care we provide. Although much yet remains to be done regarding the delivery of nursing care, we cannot ignore the pressing issues that can be resolved only through effective collaboration with other disciplines. The time is right for advancing nursing quality assurance to the next level. As we continue to enhance our impact at the bedside, we must strengthen our efforts to integrate the circle of practitioners simultaneously providing care into our pursuit of quality improvement.

REFERENCES

Crosby, P. (1979). *Quality is free*. New York: The Free Press.
Devereux, P. (1981). Does joint practice work? *Journal of Nursing Administration*, 11(6), 39-43.
Ishikawa, K. (1985). *What is total quality control? The Japanese way*. Englewood Cliffs, NJ: Prentice-Hall.

Joint Commission on Accreditation of Healthcare Organizations. (1990). *The Joint Commission's Agenda for Change; Stimulating continual improvement in the quality of care* (Agenda for Change packet). Chicago: Author.

Juran, J. M. (1988). *Juran on planning for quality*. New York: The Free Press.

Knaus, W. A., Draper, E., Wagner, D., & Zimmerman Y. (1986). An evaluation of outcome from intensive care in major medical centers. *Annals of Internal Medicine, 104*, 410-418.

Kohles, M. K., & Barry, P. L. (1989). Clinical laboratory and nursing personnel: Collaboration in improving patient care. *Journal of Nursing Quality Assurance, 3*(2), 1-10.

Peters, T. (1987). *Thriving on chaos*. New York: Harper & Row.

Puta, D. F. (1989). Nurse physician collaboration toward quality. *Journal of Nursing Quality Assurance, 3*(2), 11-18

Walton, M. (1986). *The Deming management method*. New York: Dodd, Mead, & Co.

Weiss, S. J., & Davis, H. P. (1985). Validity and reliability of the collaborative practice scales. *Nursing Research, 34*, 299-305.

CHAPTER 4

Measures of Quality

Diane L. Gardner

This chapter provides an overview of current measures of nursing quality and highlights issues in the measurement of nursing care quality. Driven by cost containment, quality of care has emerged as a corollary concern. Measurement of quality depends on the definition of quality. For the measurement of quality, it is conceptually important to distinguish quality assessment from quality assurance. The development and setting of standards also are important aspects of the process of measuring nursing care quality. The measurement of quality has become a research priority for the 1990s. This trend will dovetail with the development of uniform minimum data sets, nursing informatics, and the emphasis on total quality management and patient outcomes assessment.

You'll know it when you see it. That's how you measure the quality of health care services. This view reflects the belief of many nurses. Nevertheless, a body of knowledge about quality of care and quality assurance is being developed. The measurement and evaluation of quality, however, have remained complex and elusive. How do we measure quality? The word itself is abstract and often ambiguous. Does quality connote fine workmanship, artistic design, exclusive pricing, or amenities and fancy packaging? Is the target called *quality* constantly

The University of Iowa, Iowa City, IA 52242.

Series on Nursing Administration — Volume III, 1992

moving and therefore hard to grasp, or is quality merely a matter of individual intuition, perception, and judgment?

The purpose of this chapter is to identify controversies, questions, and issues surrounding the context within which measures of quality must be developed. Within that framework will be a discussion of instruments used in the assessment of the quality of health care. The assessment of quality will be differentiated from the evaluation of quality, and the use of standards will be discussed.

THE COST VERSUS QUALITY ISSUE

Historically, nursing pioneered in the assessment and assurance of quality nursing and health care through Florence Nightingale's documented use of standards (1858) to assess care provided to the military (Lang & Clinton, 1984b). It was not until the past two decades, however, that a renewed interest in quality assessment and quality assurance developed. Wyszewianski (1988) noted that interest in quality in the late 1960s had its origin in the rapid growth of health care expenditures. With the continued rise in health care costs, the interest in quality continues.

Precipitated by the Medicare program's radical shift to prospective reimbursement, a major current national health care theme is cost containment. Under the earlier cost-based reimbursement system, provision of maximum services was encouraged and nurses defined quality in terms of maximum care regardless of cost. Meanwhile, skyrocketing health care expenditures initiated a concern among policy makers and others as to whether the rising levels of spending were producing commensurate improvements in health (Lohr, 1988). The Medicare program's response to rising costs intensified competition in health care and created incentives to underprovide certain services. The fear that prospective payment would lead to a decline in the quality of care generated renewed interest in initiatives to ensure quality (Ginsberg & Hammons, 1988; LoGerfo, 1990). For example, both the medical treatment effectiveness program and patient outcomes research teams are supported by the Agency for Health Care Policy and Research (Salive, Mayfield, & Weisman, 1990). Achieving the delicate balance between cost and quality is a major challenge for nursing and other health care professions.

To achieve this balance, the first response in health care focused on preserving and monitoring rather than on improving quality (Wyszewianski, 1988). The widespread need for reassurance that quality would not be allowed to decline as a result of cost reduction created a pressing demand for measures of quality that were readily obtained and easily understood.

The current response incorporates a focus on customer satisfaction and on unit-based and interdisciplinary quality assurance coupled with organization-wide continuous quality improvement. Driven by consumerism and changes in health care financing, the Deming method and total quality management are being adopted in many health care settings (Darr, 1989; McLaughlin & Kaluzny, 1990).

Omachonu (1990) noted that quality consists of two interdependent parts: quality in fact and quality in perception. Quality in fact means meeting one's own expectations or conforming to standards. Quality in perception means meeting the customers' expectations. Both must be identified, defined, measured, and evaluated. Although perfect measures do not exist, considerable research has focused on measuring the quality of health care.

Definition of Quality

Any discussion of the measures of quality must address the core dilemma surrounding definition. To measure quality of care we must first identify what the purpose of that care is. Donabedian (1988) noted that the objective is an achievable state of health. Thus the purpose of health care is to move the patient from one given state of health to another. According to the Joint Commission on Accreditation of Healthcare Organizations (Joint Commission), quality of patient care is defined as the degree to which patient care services increase the probability of desired patient outcomes and reduce the probability of undesired outcomes, given the current state of knowledge (Accreditation Manual for Hospitals, 1990).

To judge the quality of the interaction between the provider and caregiver, three components must be identified: the state of the patient when caregivers become involved, the processes and structures used by the caregivers, and the state to which the patient is moved. The following diagram is a schematic representation of this interaction:

	Process	
Input	————————	Output
	Structure	
(Patient condition)		(Outcomes) (Patient condition)

Note that for nursing, it is possible to have a situation in which the input is a terminal condition and the output is a pain-free death.

Part of the ambiguity in the conceptual formulation of quality with use of this scheme is that quality reflects a desired change in the patient's initial condition (input). Thus, if there is not an initial comprehensive assessment, the ability to objectively identify changes in the output is compromised. Further ambiguity stems from comparison of the achieved outcome with the desired or ideal outcome. The desired outcome presumably is the patient's to determine. Many instances occur, however, in which other individuals involved with the process will disagree as to what is a good, appropriate, or desirable outcome. The caregiver, different family members, or even the state may take a different view. An ethical question arises when someone must, or feels an obligation to, override the patient's desires and decide on a different outcome. Thus, central to the concept of quality is a delineation of the definition of quality and who decides the desired outcomes. Selection of measures of quality reflects these decisions and involves the translation of an abstract definition of quality into specific standards and criteria that indicate appropriate outcomes to judge quality.

Quality cannot be measured until it is first defined and outcomes specified. However, the meaning of quality, as well as the desired outcomes, is variable and may change with time and circumstance. Consistency may be supplied by means of an accepted model. Donabedian (1966, 1980, 1982, 1985, 1988) established the basic health care vocabulary and concepts currently used in health care. He noted (1980) that the balance of health benefits and harms to the patient is the essential core of a definition of quality. Thus care is of high quality insofar as it contributes to the patient's health and well-being (Ginsberg & Hammons, 1988). Emphasis on the patient has provoked an ongoing debate about whether it is more important to measure outcomes than process or structure. It is clear that measurement of all three aspects—structure, process, and outcomes—is needed. As a practical matter, Donabedian (1985) pointed out that if outcomes are adverse, then poor quality is presumed and the process of care is reviewed to determine if it was deficient. Although positive outcomes do not guarantee a quality process in practice, positive outcomes are not reviewed, whereas negative outcomes serve to flag the review of process.

Donabedian (1966) classified quality of care studies into those that evaluated the components of structure, process, or outcome. He further developed the area of process (1980) by classifying the activities of care into the technical aspect, the interpersonal aspect, and the amenities of care. The technical aspect refers to the knowledge and skill of the provider in the scientific principles of care. The interpersonal aspect refers to the art of being responsive and attentive in interactions with the patient. The amenities refer to how appealing, comfortable, and private are the facilities in which care is provided. For the process of care to be truly superior, all three aspects should be of high quality. It is not necessarily true, however, that high quality in one aspect implies or ensures high quality in another (Brook & Avery, 1976).

It generally is agreed that quality has a multifaceted nature (Davis, 1987) and that there is no single definition of quality of medical care (Donabedian, 1980). Therefore there is no single measure of quality and no one composite index of quality of health care (Davis, 1987).

EVALUATION VERSUS ASSESSMENT OF QUALITY

It is important to distinguish between quality assessment and quality assurance. Quality assessment is limited to the measurement of quality. Quality assurance builds on the preceding assessment by taking evaluative action to ensure a designated level of quality (Lang & Clinton, 1984b).

Evaluation, however, involves value judgments about the attainment of goals or standards as perceived by the evaluator. Therefore the evaluation of quality requires the identification of standards. Although individuals may give different weights and values to any outcome, there has to be some agreement in terms of expected standards. To distinguish between evaluation and assessment, concepts such as standards, quality, and effectiveness need to be clearly defined. To determine if standards are met, an instrument is needed to measure the level of care accomplished (Van Maanen, 1984).

Donabedian (1980) has discussed the recurring confusion between determining efficacy and assessing quality. Determining efficacy of a procedure or intervention involves ascertaining before the fact if, under well-controlled and ideal circumstances, the intervention can reliably produce the desired effect or outcome. This is an attempt to answer the question: is this the right thing to do? Quality assessment, however, is performed after the fact to determine for a specific case whether an efficacious intervention was selected and carried out with skill and competence. The relevant question is: was the right thing done, and was it done "right"? Studies of quality require preestablished knowledge of which intervention is efficacious for each case (Wyszewianski, 1988). An incomplete knowledge base can lead to confusion if one attempts to simultaneously assess the therapeutic value of an intervention and determine the skill with which it was prescribed and performed. Thus measurement of quality (quality assessment) is different from the evaluation of quality (quality assurance).

For nursing, a major controversy surrounds the question of evaluating the effects on patient outcomes. If the patient "owns" the outcomes of care, are there nurse-sensitive patient outcomes, and what are they? How do we evaluate outcomes on which multiple health care providers have an influence? Separating and evaluating these complex and interdependent relationships will be the challenge of the future.

MEASURES OF QUALITY

Measures of quality of health care can be categorized in three areas: medical care, hospital care, and nursing care. Quality has been measured from the perspective of the provider, the organization, and the patient. Davis (1987) noted that despite the large body of literature on quality assurance and utilization review since the mid-1970s, the conceptualization and measurement instrumentation of health care quality had not progressed much beyond that of the early 1970s.

This was true until the late 1980s when the conceptual base for patient outcomes began to emerge. Initiatives at the federal level, including the new Agency for Health Care Policy and Research, sparked a research interest in developing the patient outcomes knowledge base. The medical outcomes study (MOS) (Tarlov et al., 1989) introduced a conceptual framework that identified major study variables, or key features, of medical care that are associated with patient outcomes. The focus of allied work in nursing is attempting to identify nurse-sensitive patient outcomes. Work on identifying measures of patient outcomes will be a major thrust of quality research in the next decade.

Measures of Medical Care

The bulk of the empirical work on measures of quality is related to medical (physician) care. Quality is defined by structure (characteristics of providers and the physical and organizational setting), process (technical competence plus interpersonal aspects), or outcomes (patient results of palliation, control of illness, cure, or rehabilitation). The classic list of medical outcome measures is death, disease, disability, discomfort, and dissatisfaction. The most common measures used are mortality and morbidity rates. There are those, including Lohr (1988), who prefer the positive counterparts of survival rates: states of physiologic, functional, and emotional health; and satisfaction. Other medical indicators of quality care include surgical complications, readmissions or reoperations, physiologic variables, disability days, infant and maternal mortality, life expectancy, health status measures, and patient satisfaction measures. The MOS' conceptual framework identified variables related to the structure of care (system, provider, and patient characteristics), the process of care (technical and interpersonal style), and outcomes (clinical end points, functional status, general well-being, and satisfaction with care) (Tarlov et al., 1989).

A number of health status indexes have been developed to measure functional disability and handicap, psychologic health, social health, pain, quality of life, life satisfaction, and general health (McDowell & Newell, 1987). Three well-known measures of overall health status with good reliability and validity are the Sickness Impact Profile (Gilson et al., 1975), the Quality of Well-Being Scale (Kaplan, Bush, & Berry, 1976), and the General Health Ratings Index (Davies & Ware, 1981; Read, Quinn, & Hoefer, 1987). Lohr (1988) noted that health status measures now are used primarily for health services research rather than for quality assessment or quality assurance, although they show promise as tools for quality evaluation in situations in which established links between process and outcomes are present.

Measures of Hospital Care

Measures of quality of hospital care can be focused on structure, process, or outcome. In the past, accreditation standards of the Joint Commission focused on structure and process measures. Patient satisfaction has been used as an indicator of quality of care to assess the technical and interpersonal aspects of both structure and process components. The most consistent finding is that characteristics of the provider or organization that make the care more personal are associated with higher levels of patient satisfaction (Cleary & McNeil, 1988). In one study, patient satisfaction with nursing care was a major determinant of satisfaction with a hospital stay (Abramowitz, Cote, & Berry, 1987).

The most commonly used measures of hospital care quality still are mortality and morbidity rates. Hospital mortality rates are simple, understandable measures, despite being problematic indicators of quality (Wyszewianski, 1988). They are used because patient outcomes are immensely complex to construct, mortality rates are a nonintrusive measure, and unexpected deaths are considered a sentinel event and thus an indicator that quality may have been compromised. The issue is whether the factor of avoidable death is a useful and valid outcome indicator or whether it should serve only as a screen (Lohr, 1988). With the current focus on patient outcome measures, measures of hospital mortality are not considered to be either specific or sensitive enough for quality assessment and quality assurance (Ginsberg & Hammons, 1988). The current focus of quality improvement tends to focus on the contributions of physicians and avoids recognizing the contributions of nonphysician providers and organizational processes on patient outcomes (Laffel & Blumenthal, 1989). A recent survey of chief executive officers, however, identified nursing care as the most significant factor in providing high quality care (Koska, 1989; Omachonu, 1990). As hospitals implement total quality management programs, measures of quality will be needed to evaluate the effects of change in organizational structure and function.

Measures of Nursing Care

Measures of quality of nursing care can be traced back to the 1950s. For example, Aydelotte and Tener (1960) and Aydelotte (1962) developed outcome criteria and were able to show significant relationships between nursing activities and in-service education on the one hand and patient welfare on the other. Lang and Clinton (1984a) reviewed nursing research on the assessment of quality of nursing care up to 1982 and found that in the studies devoted solely to instrument development and testing, 45% used either existing tools for measuring quality of nursing care or quality indicators developed in other disciplines. The majority of these tools were developed in the 1960s and 1970s. Among the major instruments are eight tools (identified in Table 4-1): three to measure nursing functions, two to measure nursing competency, two to measure nursing outcomes, and one to measure patient satisfaction. These valid and reliable measures represent the research effort focused on the development of criteria-based, process-oriented tools that can be used across

TABLE 4-1   Nursing Measures of Quality

Component measured	Instrument name	Author and source*
Nursing functions	Nursing audit	Phaneuf, 1976
	Quality patient care scale (QUALPACS)	Wandelt & Ager, 1974
	Rush-Medicus system	Haussmann et al., 1974
		Jelinck et al., 1974
		Hegyvary & Haussmann, 1976
Nursing competency	Slater nursing competencies rating scale	Wandelt & Stewart, 1975
	Schwirian six-dimensional scale of nursing performance	Schwirian, 1978, 1981
Nursing outcomes	Criterion measures of nursing care quality	Horn & Swain, 1978
	Sickness impact profile	Gilson et al., 1975
		Read et al., 1987
Patient satisfaction	Patient satisfaction instrument	Hinshaw & Atwood, 1982

* See chapter reference list for complete citation.

patient populations and among various health care settings. The goal of the work in the 1960s and 1970s was to establish a basis for national standards of nursing excellence (Lang & Clinton, 1984a; Phaneuf & Wandelt, 1982).

The Phaneuf nursing audit (Phaneuf, 1972) is designed to evaluate overall quality of care by focusing on the process of care as it is reflected in a retrospective chart audit. The tool was constructed by subdividing seven basic functions of nursing care into 50 components. For each component there is an assessment made on a 5-point scale ranging from excellent to unsafe. Scores are summed, and a subtotal for each function and a grand total for nursing care as a whole are derived. Although Phaneuf (1976) noted that development of the nursing audit began in 1952, scale development, reliability, and validity are not reported. Maibusch (1984) indicated that questions about the reliability and validity of this tool have not been satisfactorily answered. The tool does not use outcomes as measurable changes in the patient's status.

The quality patient care scale (QUALPACS) (Wandelt & Ager, 1974) is derived from the Slater competency scale and is designed to globally measure quality of care in any setting at the time care is being given. This 68-item scale is arranged into six subsections and provides a mean score.

Use of this scale requires direct observation of a patient. It designates the use of a controlled random selection of patients to evaluate unit-level quality of care. Good reliability and validity have been reported in the results of six studies in which the tool was used.

The Rush-Medicus system (Haussmann, Hegyvary, Newman, & Bishop, 1974) is a global measure of quality of care based on the nursing process. It was developed through a three-phase research study. About 250 criteria are divided into two parts, each of which has six classes (objectives) with 28 categories (subobjectives) distributed among the classes. Subobjectives are a series of specific criteria related to a specific subject. The authors suggest that 10% of 1 month's patient census be reviewed when the system is used. This instrument received extensive reliability and validity testing. The tool is used to relate adherence to the nursing process to expected outcomes.

Among the instruments designed to measure nursing performance, the Slater nursing competencies rating scale (Wandelt & Stewart, 1975) is an 84-item scale designed to identify quality of care through nurse observation. This instrument is used retrospectively. The items are arranged into six subsections, each with 7 to 18 criteria. This well-validated scale has had extensive testing, and its use is reported in six studies.

The Schwirian six-dimensional scale of nursing performance (Schwirian, 1978, 1981) consists of 52 rating-scale items grouped into six subscales to measure nursing performance in a variety of practice settings. The scale was developed as a part of a national project on nursing competencies, and good reliability and validity have been reported. McCloskey (McCloskey & McCain, 1988) used this instrument in a recent study of nurse performance.

Horn and Swain (1978) studied a method of measuring patient health status in terms of outcomes of care influenced by nursing. They developed an instrument based on Orem's theory, which includes 539 validated criterion measures of nursing care. Reliability and validity are reported, although this instrument was tested only partially. The instrument has not been used widely (Maibusch, 1984); however, it shows promise as a unique tool to measure functional health status and its relationship to nursing process.

The Sickness impact profile (Gilson et al., 1975) has 136 statements organized into 12 categories that represent components of health. It is a behaviorally based measure of sickness-related dysfunction and includes both physical and psychosocial dimensions. This instrument has been tested and exhibits good overall reliability and validity. It has been used more for medical than for nursing research.

Hinshaw and Atwood's 18-item patient satisfaction instrument (1982) was developed through a series of studies and contains a Likert-type summated rating scale with three dimensions of patient satisfaction. This scale, like the LaMonica-Oberst patient satisfaction scale (LaMonica, Oberst, Madea, & Wolf, 1986), was developed from the Risser (1975) scale through modification and testing. Good reliability and validity are reported. This instrument has been extensively tested and used.

Jacquerye (1984) critiqued some of the preceding methods of evaluating quality of care and found the Phaneuf (1976) nursing audit an easy and economical method for quality assurance. She found the Wandelt and Ager (1974) QUALPACS scale easy to use but problematic for applying corrective action in the practice setting. The Rush-Medicus system (Haussmann et al., 1974) was found to be difficult to apply in the practice setting. The Horn and Swain (1978) method was noted to be designed for easy use by staff nurses, however, some of the criterion measures are not specific to nursing but can be influenced by other disciplines.

There are many other measures of quality reported in the literature. One nursing service administration resource laboratory has gathered more than 82 instruments related to measuring patient outcomes (Clougherty et al., 1991). Books on quality measurement also are beginning to appear (Spath, 1989).

The challenge for the future will be to identify the variables relevant to the study of quality in nursing, to test and establish appropriate measures for these variables, and then to investigate the interrelationships among cost, quality, organizational variables, decision-making processes, provider satisfaction, and patient outcomes. Initial research includes the investigation of the implied meaning of quality (Jackson-Frankl, 1990), the link between cost and quality in nurse staffing decisions (Behner, Fogg, Fournier, Frankenbach, & Robertson, 1990), and the effect of DRG reimbursement on patient acuity, length of stay, and quality of nursing care (Van Hoesen & Ericksen, 1990).

Current Focus in Measurement

In the 1980s, the focus of evaluation efforts shifted in an attempt to develop and refine measures of quality that are centered on the structure aspect of costs (financial resources) and the outcome aspect of patient outcomes. Efforts to ascertain the cost of nursing services, usually on the basis of patient acuity or patient classification systems, are aimed at demonstrating how to reduce costs while maintaining or improving quality of care. Thus the focus is on efficiency in the technical aspects of care. As nursing tackles the issue of knowing what it will cost to do certain activities, it becomes important to determine the cost-quality ratio per outcome. This, in turn, may facilitate a systematic review of the utilization of nursing time, effort, and activities and may stimulate additional research on nursing effectiveness and patient outcomes that will include an elaboration and refinement of measurement tools.

The recent emphasis on measuring quality of care has uncovered the gap in availability of standardized data-collection measures and data bases for comparing the effectiveness of care across units, institutions, and regions. Thus the movement for uniform minimum data sets is beginning to emerge as a practice issue. Sovie (1988) and Werley, Lang, and Westlake (1986) have argued for the establishment of a nursing minimum data set, with uniform definitions and elements used by all hospitals and investigators to foster standardized reporting and comparisons.

Investigation of measures of quality in nursing has intensified in the area of patient outcomes. A two-volume collection of nursing measurement tools (Strickland & Waltz, 1988; Waltz & Strickland, 1988) includes reliability and validity assessments for measuring outcomes of nursing education and practice. Volume 1 contains a collection of tools that addresses client outcomes related to illness, wellness, community care, and quality of care; volume 2 contains a collection of tools that addresses provider-centered outcomes such as role socialization, continuing education, clinical competency, and student assessment. Two measures of quality of care included in volume 1 are Van Servellen's individualized care index (1988), a measure of nursing functions, and Erikson's nursing care questionnaire (1988), a measure of patient satisfaction. These tools have documented reliability and validity and appear usable in the clinical setting. Another tool that appears useful for the measurement of clinical outcomes is the Patunk indicators of nursing care (PINC) instrument (Majesky, Brester, & Nishio, 1978). It has been used to evaluate the relationship between patient outcomes and various nursing inputs (Lamb-Mechanick, 1989).

Little research has been conducted in the areas of home care and long-term care, although a few measurement instruments have been developed. Rinke (1987) has compiled a volume of outcome measures in home care, and Lalonde (1986, 1987) has gathered seven outcome scales with reliability, validity, and usability rating. The rapid disability rating scale (Linn, 1967) and the cumulative illness rating scale (Linn, Linn, & Gurel, 1968) are two measures used for research in long-term care (Linn, Gurel, & Linn, 1977).

Overall, there is a considerable body of knowledge related to measures of quality. Reliable and valid measures of many aspects of nursing care are available for researchers and clinicians. The practicality and usability of these tools vary. Most of these instruments have been used primarily by researchers rather than by practitioners in the clinical setting. General awareness about the existence of a large number of these tools has not been widespread. This is due in part to the slowness with which research has been utilized in clinical practice and in part to the service sector's need for simple measurement instruments that are easy to apply in the practice setting.

STANDARDS AND QUALITY MEASUREMENTS

The development and setting of standards of quality are the first and most basic steps in the process of conducting quality assurance activities. The overall process includes setting standards, monitoring practice, evaluating identified practice problems, and resolving those practice problems (Schroeder, 1988). The development and use of standards are emphasized in the literature about quality of care, because standards are used to derive criteria against which care is measured for quality assurance purposes. Usually the criteria that accompany a standard are derived from quality assessment studies if they are available (Taylor, 1974). Patterson (1988) defined quality as a numerical ratio that represents the degree of adherence between the nursing standard of care and observed patient outcomes. Thus quality comes to mean that degree of compliance with generally recognized standards of good nursing practice and the achievement of anticipated patient outcomes as measured against the standards of care.

In order to have a system to evaluate the quality of nursing care, there must be criteria that measure the results or outcomes of care. The knowledge base on which to develop such criteria is still weak. There is lack of agreement about content needed in a minimum data set to establish norms and form a basis for comparing effectiveness (Taylor, 1974). Schroeder (1988) noted that the term *standards* carries with it an incredible confusion. Patterson (1988) reviewed the literature and found evidence of such confusion. She identified and defined two terms that need clarification: standard of care and standard of practice. A standard of care focuses on the recipient of care (the patient), and a standard of practice focuses on the provider of care (the nurse). A standard of care is written in patient outcomes, whereas a standard of practice is written about the nursing process. This echoes the Donabedian theme of process and outcome as two components of the quality-of-care triad.

Besides the confusion of terms, there is a proliferation of standards developed by multiple discrete groups of nurses. Often each agency develops its own. Standards come from different sources and are based on frameworks as diverse as nursing process, health care needs, body systems, or the process of care. They are then used in agencies, with philosophic frameworks derived from nursing diagnoses, developmental stages, or medical diagnoses. The challenge is to organize and integrate these standards with the philosophy and care delivery method (Schroeder, 1988). It is clear that there is little uniformity among the types and uses of standards of care. Moreover, there is no unanimity within the profession concerning the desired degree of uniformity.

Although evaluation standards should be flexible, a measurement instrument is required to determine the level of care that has been delivered (Van Maanen, 1984). With the current national concern for demonstrating that quality care has been delivered, measures of quality are critical. Yet the state of the art is such that definitions are confusing and measurement tools not widely tested nor used in practice.

An unresolved issue relates to autonomy and control over practice. Who will set the standards? Will they be set by practicing staff nurses, nurse administrators, the organizations in which nurses practice, nursing organizations, the Joint Commission, or legislative or regulatory bodies? Nurse researchers will argue for more time to thoroughly investigate and test the data base. Nurses in practice will argue for understandable and usable tools that validly measure quality. Organizations and regulatory bodies will argue for immediate data, often seeking only evidence that minimum requirements are met. Consumers will argue for an array of simple measures of satisfaction and quality.

Thus the measurement of quality will be an amalgam of which definitions are chosen, who defines the aspects of quality to be measured, and what outcomes are considered desirable or valuable. Standards and criteria are alleged to be the domain of the professionals, and nursing has much work to do if it is to provide leadership to consumers and other groups that have a legitimate interest in defining quality health care.

CONCLUSION

Nurse administrators actively deal with the delicate balance of cost and quality. They must respond to patients, families, providers, organizations, and regulatory agencies, whose needs and desires often appear to conflict. How nurse administrators creatively balance these forces sets the tone for the perception of quality of care in their organizations.

If it is true that anything that exists can be measured and the ability to measure depends on the sophistication of the measurement instrument, then quality can be measured. Nurse administrators need to grapple with the core questions of who decides, who defines, whose needs are met, and at what level are those needs met? Should quality be defined as just meeting requirements? Should we set expectations that quality be defined as an ideal situation? Or should quality be defined as outcomes that can be achieved, given the resources available? Should the caregivers' perspective prevail? Should standards be determined by professionals or by organizations? Should input, structure, process, and outcomes be emphasized equally or differentially? How much importance should be placed on each? Many of these questions have no absolute answers. The decisions made in practice, however, will shape professional priorities for action and will determine how resources are used to achieve quality care.

As the measurement of quality of care becomes a research priority, nurse administrators must ask whether previous research activities have missed their mark. Do the results of research studies reflect the perspective of the patient and family, as well as that of the provider, in regard to the perception of quality care? Has the measurement of quality produced results that can be used to evaluate and modify management and care delivery systems? Are we using this information to change our practice and to change the health care system?

Nurse administrators should take an active role in identifying, examining, and defining what is absolutely critical for nurses to do to provide quality health care to patients. This applies both to individual cases and to groups of patients. Because there are multiple influences simultaneously involved in improving a patient's health status, nurses are faced with the problem of determining the changes that are attributable to nursing care. Acceptance of the idea that quality outcomes extend along a continuum, as opposed to an absolute standard, can result in an understanding of the dynamic and multidimensional nature of quality care.

Quality care is a holistic concept with many dimensions. Although measures are available for some of these dimensions, more refinement is needed to produce convenient measures with simple formats that achieve easily displayed data and trend measurement. Performance aspects to be measured include technical skill and competence, interpersonal elements, input health status, amenities, convenience and access, continuity of care, outcomes, and patient and provider satisfaction. The quest for quality raises an array of intriguing questions but ensures no simple solutions.

REFERENCES

Abramowitz, S., Cote, A., & Berry, E. (1987). Analyzing patient satisfaction: a multianalytic approach. *Quality Review Bulletin, 13*, 122-130.

Accreditation Manual for Hospitals (1990). Chicago: Joint Commission on Accreditation of Heathcare Organizations.

Aydelotte, M. (1962). The use of patient welfare as a criterion measure. *Nursing Research, 11*(1), 10-14.

Aydelotte, M., & Tener, M. (1960). *An investigation of the relation between nursing activity and patient welfare.* Iowa City: State University of Iowa.

Behner, K., Fogg, L., Fournier, L., Frakenbach, J., & Robertson, S. (1990). Nursing resource management: Analyzing the relationship between costs and quality in staffing decisions. *Health Care Management Review, 15*(4), 63-71.

Brook, R., & Avery, A. (1976). *Quality assessment: Issues of definition and measurement.* Santa Monica, CA: The Rand Corp.

Cleary, P., & McNeil, B. (1988). Patient satisfaction as an indicator of quality care. *Inquiry, 25*, 25-36.

Clougherty, J., McCloskey, J. C., Johnson, M., Casula, M., Gardner, D., Kelly, K., Maas, M., Delaney, C., & Blegen, M. (1991). Creating a resource data base for nursing service administration. *Computers in Nursing, 9*(4), 69-74.

Darr, K. (1989). Applying the Deming method in hospitals. I. *Hospital Topics, 67*(6), 4-5.

Darr, K. (1989). Applying the Deming method in hospitals. II. *Hospital Topics, 68*(1), 4-6.

Davis, F. (1987). Quality of health care measurement: A research priority. *Health Care Financing Review* (annual suppl.), 1-3.

Donabedian, A. (1966). Evaluating the quality of medical care. *Milbank Memorial Fund Quarterly, 44*, 166-206.

Donabedian, A. (1980). *Explorations in quality assessment and monitoring: The definition of quality and approaches to its assessment* (Vol. 1). Ann Arbor, MI: Health Administration Press.

Donabedian, A. (1982). *Explorations in quality assessment and monitoring: The criteria and standards of quality* (Vol. 2). Ann Arbor, MI: Health Administration Press.

Donabedian, A. (1985). *Explorations in quality assessment and monitoring: The methods and findings of quality assessment and monitoring* (Vol. 3). Ann Arbor, MI: Health Administration Press.

Donabedian, A. (1988). Quality assessment and assurance: unity of purpose, diversity of means. *Inquiry, 25*(1), 173-192.

Erikson, L. (1988). Measuring patient satisfaction with nursing care: A magnitude estimation approach. In C. Waltz & O. Strickland (Eds.), *Measurement of nursing outcomes: Measuring client outcomes.* Vol. 1. New York: Springer.

Gilson, B., Gilson, J., Bergner, M., Bobbitt, R., Kressel, S., Pollard, W., & Vesselago, M. (1975). The sickness impact profile: Development of an outcome measure of health care. *American Journal of Public Health, 65,* 1304-1310.

Ginsberg, P., & Hammons, G. (1988). Competition and the quality of care: The importance of information. *Inquiry, 25,* 108-115.

Haussmann, R., Hegyvary, S., Newman, F., & Bishop, A. (1974) Monitoring quality of nursing care. *Health Services Research, 9,* 135-148.

Hegyvary, S., & Haussmann, R. (1976). Correlates of the quality of nursing care. *Journal of Nursing Administration, 6*(9), 18-21.

Hinshaw, A. S., & Atwood, J. R. (1982). A patient satisfaction instrument: Precision by replication. *Nursing Research, 31,* 170-175.

Horn, B., & Swain, M. (1978). *Criterion measures of nursing care quality* (Final report US DHEW). Hyattsville, MD: National Center for Health Services Research (NTIS No. PB-287 449/3GA).

Jackson-Frankl, K. (1990). The language and meaning of quality. *Nursing Administration Quarterly, 14*(3), 52-65.

Jacquerye, A. (1984). Choosing an appropriate method of quality assurance. *Recent Advances in Nursing, 10,* 107-120.

Jelinek, R., Haussmann, R., Hegyvary, S., & Newman, J. (1974). *A methodology for monitoring quality of nursing care (DHEW Publication No. 76-25).* Washington, DC: U.S. Government Printing Office.

Kaplan, R., Bush, J., & Berry, C. (1976). Health status: Types of validity and the index of well-being. *Health Services Research, 11,* 448-507.

Koska, M. (1989). Quality—Thy name is nursing care, CEOs say. *Hospitals, 63*(3), 32.

Laffel, G., & Blumenthal, D. (1989). The case for using industrial quality management science in health care organizations. *Journal of the American Medical Association, 262,* 2869-2873.

Lalonde, B. (1986). *Quality Assurance Manual of the Home Care Association of Washington.* Edmonds, WA: The Home Care Association of Washington.

Lalonde, B. (1987). The general symptom distress scales: A home care outcome measure. *Quality Review Bulletin, 13,* 243-250.

Lamb-Mechanick, D. (1989). Usefulness of a patient outcome instrument to evaluate nursing resource allocation. *Journal of Nursing Administration, 19*(11), 3.

LaMonica, E., Oberst, M., Madea, A., & Wolf, R. (1986). Development of a patient satisfaction scale. *Research in Nursing & Health, 9*(1), 43-50.

Lang, N., & Clinton, J. (1984a). Assessment of quality of nursing care. In H. Werley & J. Fitzpatrick (Eds.). *Annual review of nursing research* (Vol. 2). New York: Springer.

Lang, N., & Clinton, J. (1984b). Quality assurance: The idea and its development in the United States. *Recent Advances in Nursing, 10,* 69-88.

Linn, B., Linn, M., & Gurel, L. (1968). Cumulative illness rating scale. *Journal of the American Geriatrics Society, 16,* 622-626.

Linn, M. (1967). A rapid disability rating scale. *Journal of the American Geriatrics Society*, *15*, 211-214.

Linn, M., Gurel, L., & Linn, B. (1977). Patient outcome as a measure of quality of nursing home care. *American Journal of Public Health*, *67*, 337-344.

LoGerfo, J. (1990). The prospective payment system and quality: No skeletons in the closet. *Journal of the American Medical Association*, *264*, 1995-1996.

Lohr, K. (1988). Outcome measurement: Concepts and questions, *Inquiry*, *25*(1), 37-50.

Maibusch, R. (1984). Evolution of quality assurance for nursing in hospitals. In P. Schroeder & R. Maibusch (Eds.). *Nursing Quality Assurance*. Rockville, MD: Aspen Systems Corp.

Majesky, S., Brester, M., & Nishio, K. (1978). Development of a research tool: Patient indicators of nursing care. *Nursing Research*, *27*, 356-371.

McCloskey, J., & McCain, B. (1988). Variables related to nurse performance. *Image*, *20*, 203-207.

McDowell, I., & Newell, C. (1987). *Measuring health: A guide to rating scales and questionnaires*. New York: Oxford University Press.

McLaughlin, C., & Kaluzny, A. (1990). Total quality management in health: Making it work. *Health Care Management Review*, *15*(3), 7-14.

Nightingale, F. (1858). *Notes on matters affecting the health, efficiency, and hospital administration of the British army*. London: Harrison & Sons.

Omachonu, V. K. (1990). Quality of care and the patient: New criteria for evaluation. *Health Care Management Review*, *15*(4), 43-50.

Patterson, C. (1988). Standards for patient care: The Joint Commission focus on nursing quality assurance. *Nursing Clinics of North America*, *23*, 625-638.

Phaneuf, M. (1972). *The nursing audit: Profile for excellence*. New York: Appleton-Century-Crofts.

Phaneuf, M. (1976). *The nursing audit: Self-regulation in nursing practice*. New York: Appleton-Century-Crofts.

Phaneuf, M., & Wandelt, M. (1982). Three methods of process-oriented nursing evaluation. *Quality Review Bulletin (Special edition on nursing review: Criteria for evaluation and analysis of patient care)*, 32-38.

Read, J., Quinn, R., & Hoefer, M. (1987). Measuring overall health: An evaluation of three important approaches. *Journal of Chronic Diseases*, *40*(Suppl. 1), 7S-21S.

Rinke, L. (1987). *Outcome measures in home care: Vol 1. Research*. (Publication No. 21-2194). New York: National League for Nursing.

Risser, N. (1975). Development of an instrument to measure patient satisfaction with nurses and nursing care in primary settings. *Nursing Research*, *24*(1), 45-52.

Salive, M., Mayfield, J., & Weisman, N. (1990). Patient outcomes research teams and the agency for health care policy and research. *Health Services Research*, *25*, 697-708.

Schroeder, P. (1988). Directions and dilemmas in nursing quality assurance. *Nursing Clinics of North America*, *23*, 657-664.

Schwirian, P. (1978). Evaluating the performance of nurses: A multidimensional approach. *Nursing Research*, *27*, 347-351.

Schwirian, P. (1981). Toward an explanatory model of nursing performance. *Nursing Research*, *30*, 247-253.

Sovie, M. (1988). Variable costs of nursing care in hospitals. In J. Fitzpatrick, R. Taunton, & J. Benoliel (Eds.). *Annual review of nursing research*. New York: Springer.

Spath, P. (1989). *Innovations in health care quality measurement* (AHA Publication No. 169101). Chicago: American Hospital Association Publishing, Inc.

Strickland, O., & Waltz, C. (1988). *Measurement of nursing outcomes: Vol. 2. Measuring nursing performance: Practice, education, and research*. New York: Springer.

Tarlov, A., Ware, J., Greenfield, S., Nelson, E., Perrin, E., & Zubkoff, M. (1989). The medical outcomes study: An application of methods for monitoring the results of medical care. *Journal of the American Medical Association*, *262*, 925-930.

Taylor, J. (1974). Measuring the outcomes of nursing care. *Nursing Clinics of North America, 9,* 337-348.

Van Hoesen, N., & Ericksen, L. (1990). The impact of diagnosis-related groups on patient acuity, quality of care, and length of stay. *Journal of Nursing Administration, 20*(9), 20-23.

Van Maanen, H. (1984). Evaluation of nursing care: Quality of nursing evaluated within the context of health care and examined from a multinational perspective. *Recent Advances in Nursing, 10,* 3-42.

Van Servellen, G. (1988). The individualized care index. In C. Waltz & O. Strickland (Eds.). *Measurement of nursing outcomes: Measuring client outcomes* (Vol. 1). New York: Springer.

Waltz, C., & Strickland, O. (1988). *Measurement of nursing outcomes: Measuring client outcomes* (Vol. 1). New York: Springer.

Wandelt, M., & Ager, J. (1974). *Quality patient care scale.* New York: Appleton-Century-Crofts.

Wandelt, M. & Stewart, D. (1975). *Slater nursing competencies rating scale.* New York: Appleton-Century-Crofts.

Werley, H., Lang, N., & Westlake, S. (1986). Brief summary of the nursing minimum data set conference. *Nursing Management, 17*(7), 42-45.

Wyszewianski, L. (1988). Quality of care: Past achievements and future challenges. *Inquiry, 25*(1), 13-22.

CHAPTER 5

Quality in the Nineties

Marion Johnson
Joanne Comi McCloskey

Patient outcomes are an integral component of effectiveness research, which studies linkages between process and outcomes and structure and outcomes. Current initiatives in outcome measurement directed by government and private agencies are presented. The emphasis on outcome identification and measurement has implications for nursing research and practice and creates issues that must be addressed by the profession.

Health care quality is emerging as a major issue of the 1990s, but unlike the 1970s, when the focus was on improving quality, the current focus is on preserving quality (Wyszewianski, 1988). This change has resulted in an emphasis on *monitoring* quality and on developing outcomes that can serve as quality monitors. These changes stem from concern about the effects of cost-containment efforts on the quality and accessibility of health care services. This chapter briefly describes some of the changes taking place in how quality is measured, outlines current initiatives in outcomes management, and discusses the implications of current efforts for nursing.

The University of Iowa, Iowa City, IA 52242.

Series on Nursing Administration — Volume III, 1992

REDEFINING QUALITY

The focus of quality assurance efforts has shifted from structure and process indicators to outcomes of care. This shift is a direct result of the failure of a decade of cost-containment efforts. According to Aiken (1988) previous cost-containment strategies have focused on (1) increasing productivity and efficiency, (2) limiting the growth of wages and prices, and (3) reducing the amount of care provided. The greatest cost savings can be realized by reducing the amount of care provided and therein lies the current dilemma: how to reduce services and maintain quality when little is known about the relative effectiveness of treatments. Without this knowledge, the tendency has been to reduce services across the board, resulting in uncertainty about the quality and distribution of health care services among consumers, payers, and health care professionals.

To contain costs and maintain quality, information is needed about the effects of health care interventions and treatments. This need has resulted in the current emphasis on patient outcomes as measures of treatment effectiveness. The focus on effectiveness rather than on quality represents a second shift in the evaluation of health care services. Although these terms are similar, they are not identical. Health care professionals have tended to define quality in terms of efficacy — the outcomes that can be achieved when a treatment occurs under *ideal* conditions — that is, provided by the most skilled practitioner in the best possible circumstances (Lohr, 1988; Roper, Winkenwerder, Hackbarth, & Krakayer, 1988). Quality then becomes a moving target; better outcomes are potentially possible if one can improve the conditions under which the treatment is provided. This makes it difficult, if not impossible, to define and consequently to measure quality. Effectiveness, on the other hand, indicates the outcomes or benefits that actually are achieved under ordinary circumstances for typical patients (Lohr, 1988). Theoretically, effectiveness is easier to measure because it requires only the identification of achieved outcomes. The problem, of course, is developing valid, reliable outcome measures. Currently, methods and instruments for gathering and analyzing outcome data are underdeveloped (Roper et al., 1988). This inability to quantify outcomes has created problems in the study of linkages between structure and outcomes and process and outcomes, the foundation of effectiveness research.

A prime mover in the shift toward effectiveness as the measure of quality has been the federal government. The government's definition of effectiveness, however, is broader than that already described. The government viewpoint includes the necessity and appropriateness of interventions, as well as the benefits, that can be accrued at a given cost (Peters, 1989; Roper, 1988). Research that ties cost to benefits suggests how care can be reduced while maintaining acceptable levels of quality (Aiken, 1988). Determining the appropriateness and necessity of health care services requires the quantification of both costs and benefits. Although costs are relatively easy to identify, quantification of benefits depends on the identification, measurement, and analysis of outcomes of care. As the government has pushed for descriptions of the relationships among interventions, costs, and outcomes, a new language has been generated in quality assurance.

Outcomes management was coined to describe the implementation of a national data base containing information about clinical, financial, and health outcomes that can be used to describe the relationship between medical interventions and outcomes and between money and outcomes (Ellwood, 1988). As described by Ellwood, outcomes management relies on standards and guidelines to be used in selecting appropriate medical interventions, the measurement of patient function and well-being in addition to clinical outcomes, national pooling of clinical and outcome data, and analysis of the relationships between outcomes and other variables of interest, such as medical intervention or money spent. Although use of the term has expanded to include management of outcomes at the organizational as well as the national level, Ellwood's description has played a role in shaping the current emphasis on outcomes. Because outcomes are intrinsic to current definitions of effective health care, a number of initiatives directed at the description, measurement, and management of outcomes are under way.

INITIATIVES IN OUTCOME MANAGEMENT

The federal government is playing a major role in advancing patient outcomes as indicators of health care quality. In December 1989 the Agency for Health Care Policy and Research (AHCPR) was established as the successor to the National Center for Health Services Research and Health Care Technology Assessment (NCHSR). The purpose of the new agency is to enhance the quality, appropriateness, and effectiveness of health care services and to improve access to that care (AHCPR, Sept. 1990). The agency's Medical Treatment Effectiveness Program (MEDTEP) is charged with examining the effects of variations in health care practices on patient outcomes. As part of this program, practice guidelines are being formulated with the help of the professional community: "Guidelines convert science-based knowledge into clinical action in a form accessible to practitioners, thus enabling professional judgment to inform the health care provider of preferred treatment; clarify health care choices and their consequences for the patient; and link quality assurance and cost effectiveness to health care management" (AHCPR, Feb. 1990, p. 1). The government is concerned about the high cost of health care, and this newest approach to lower costs is an effort to determine whether the most expensive treatment is always warranted or even effective. Multidisciplinary panels of health care experts are convened to develop the guidelines. The first seven panels convened are exploring the following topics (AHCPR, Aug. 1990, p. 2):

- Visual impairment because of cataracts in the aging eye
- Diagnosis and treatment of benign prostatic hyperplasia
- Pain management
- Diagnosis and treatment of depressed outpatients in primary care settings
- Delivery of comprehensive care in sickle cell disease
- Prediction, prevention, and early treatment of pressure sores in adults
- Urinary incontinence in the adult

Three of the panels (on pain, pressure sores, and urinary incontinence) are chaired or cochaired by nurses. This participation by nurses resulted from a meeting on January 31 and February 1, 1990, when AHCPR convened an ad hoc advisory panel of nurses to provide the profession's prospective on its role in the overall MEDTEP initiative. This group of 45 nursing leaders concluded that the purpose of guidelines "is to guide practice by providing linkages among diagnoses, treatments, and outcomes, and by describing the alternatives available for each patient. Guidelines provide the basis for evaluation of care and allocation of resources" (AHCPR, Feb. 1990, p. 1).

In addition to this major endeavor, the government is involved in other activities related to the establishment of outcomes. The Health Care Financing Administration (HCFA), while continuing to monitor mortality, morbidity, disability, and cost for Medicare recipients, also will analyze variations in outcomes, assess interventions, and provide feedback and education for medical practitioners (Roper et al., 1988). The establishment of the Uniform Clinical Data Set in 1987 is part of HCFA's effort to standardize clinical guidelines and to develop outcome measures. It is anticipated that Medicare coverage decisions and payment policies of the future will be guided by the findings of effectiveness research and Medicare data analysis (Roper, 1990).

Payment for nursing home and community care also may be tied to patient outcomes. The Omnibus Reconciliation Act (OBRA) of 1987 mandates the development of patient outcome measures as one component of the survey process for nursing homes participating in Medicare and Medicaid (Peters, 1989). By 1993 these measures will be part of the evaluation process used to determine funding. OBRA also imposed a number of conditions on the survey process for home care (Washington Focus, 1988). Included in the new requirements are techniques for measuring the quality of services in terms of patient outcomes.

Nongovernmental efforts also are being directed at the use of patient outcomes as measures of quality. The Joint Commission on Accreditation of Healthcare Organizations (Joint Commission) has adopted "Redefining Quality" as their agenda for the 1990s. A major thrust of the program is the identification of clinical and organizational quality indicators (O'Leary,

1987). Clinical indicators, which include outcomes of care, are being established by Joint Commission task forces for identified patient populations and clinical areas. A number of indicators are ready for testing, including those for oncology patients, trauma patients, cardiovascular patients, and obstetric patients (Joint Commission, 1989, 1990). After testing, single occurrence or rate threshold standards will be established for each of the clinical indicators (Wiltse, 1990). Hospitals will be required to collect and analyze data in relation to all clinical indicators, to explain any variance, and to describe the steps being taken to control the variance.

The Blue Cross and Blue Shield Association also is focusing on quality through its Center for Quality Healthcare. As part of its program it will be testing an Outcomes Management System (OMS) developed by Inter-Study in 10 of its Plans during 1990 (Madden, 1990). This system, designed for computerized medical records, collects data on patients' clinical condition, functional status, and satisfaction with care. The Blues have already initiated a program that screens surgical procedures with high utilization rates in six of their Plans. As health care costs continue to escalate, third-party payers can be expected to increase their requirements for information supporting the necessity and appropriateness of treatment for which they are paying.

A number of research efforts, supported by both private and public funds, are directed at the measurement of patient outcomes. One of the most comprehensive is the MOS sponsored by the Henry J. Kaiser Family Foundation, the Robert Wood Johnson Foundation, the Pew Charitable Trusts, the National Center for Health Services Research, the National Institute on Aging, the National Institute of Mental Health, the Rand Corporation, and the New England Medical Center (Greenfield, 1990). The purposes of the MOS were to develop more practical tools for monitoring patient outcomes and to relate variations in outcomes to structural and process components of physician care (Tarlov et al., 1989). The four outcome categories used in the study were clinical end points, functional status, general well-being, and satisfaction with care.

Current efforts to measure patient outcomes and determine cost effectiveness are directed primarily at the outcomes of physician care. This has occurred for a number of reasons. First, physician-directed interventions account for 80% of our health care expenditures (Grace, 1990) and consequently are a primary target for cost-effectiveness research. Second, the necessary information must be systematically recorded and available in the medical record. To date, information that meets this criterion is that related to medical diagnoses and physician-directed treatment procedures. Third is the focus of our health care system. Nationally, health care has focused on the treatment of illness that is primarily physician directed rather than on the maintenance of health that relies on a multidisciplinary approach. The current approach to effectiveness research, however, should require attention to the interventions of other health care professionals. Patient outcomes, especially those related to functional status, well-being, and satisfaction, are not achieved solely through physician intervention. The opportunity for nursing to demonstrate its contributions to health care has never been so great, nor have the challenges facing nursing been quite so important.

IMPLICATIONS FOR NURSING

For nursing interventions and outcomes to be included in the evaluation of health care, it is absolutely imperative that nurses come to some agreement about information to be systematically collected and terminology to be used in the collection process. Without such an organized body of information, all attempts to include nurse-sensitive outcomes in the evaluative process will fail. As an example, the critical indicators being developed by the Joint Commission are primarily outcomes of physician practice. As a nurse on the obstetrics task force explained, efforts to incorporate outcomes related specifically to nursing practice were not successful because the necessary information is not universally collected and retrievable from the medical record (Wiltse, 1990).

The American Nurses' Association (ANA) is working toward the development of a standardized data base for nursing in conjunction with AHCPR. As a result of the previously mentioned ad hoc advisory meeting with AHCPR and a follow-up conference in May, 1990 (O'Connor, 1990), the ANA has increased its emphasis on establishing a national nursing data base. Ongoing actions include the establishment of a steering committee on data bases by the Congress of Nursing Practice (ANA, April 30-May 1, 1990). The charge to the steering committee is (1) to propose policy and program initiatives regarding nursing classification schemes, uniform nursing data sets, and the inclusion of nursing data elements into national data bases and (2) to coordinate ANA's initiatives related to all public and private efforts regarding the development of data bases and their relationship to the development and maintenance of practice standards and guidelines and payment reform for nursing services. A second related activity concerns the gathering and cataloging of existing nursing standards. The ANA intends to "collect, catalog and analyze what information currently exists regarding nursing practice standards, practice guidelines, performance measures and review criteria" (ANA, 1990). It is quite likely that the ANA will endorse some existing efforts as part of its nursing data base work. For example, ANA is encouraging the North American Nursing Diagnosis Association (NANDA) to develop more fully its list of nursing diagnoses and to include the diagnoses of the ANA Council on Psychiatric and Mental Health Nursing, the Association of Critical Care Nurses, and the Omaha community health list. The ANA also is providing assistance to an ongoing effort at The University of Iowa to construct and validate a classification of nursing interventions (McCloskey et al., 1990). The development of data bases is a necessary and arduous first step. As work is being done on data base development, plans for implementation need to be addressed.

Implementation of a nursing data base, unless enforced by government, is in the hands of nurse administrators. Nursing only recently has recognized the need for systematic data collection, and few data bases have been available for national implementation. For those that are available, implementation has been slow. For example, the use of established nursing diagnoses is not universal in all practice settings despite the fact that a classification of nursing diagnoses has been available since the mid 1970s. The Nursing Minimum Data Set (Werley & Lang, 1988) is another attempt to organize nursing information in a systematic way. At a conference in May 1985, a group of nurse experts identified 16 variables that should be gathered systematically in all care settings. The key variables—those that describe nursing practice—were diagnoses, interventions, outcomes, and intensity of nursing care (Werley & Lang, 1988). Testing and implementation of the data set have been slow (Simpson, 1991). Two key problems are the lack of computerization in clinical nursing documentation and the lack of a classification of nursing interventions. The classification of nursing interventions is being addressed by the Iowa group, which, in June 1990, received funding for the work from the National Center for Nursing Research.

These efforts for organizing and collecting nursing information systematically must be supported by nurse administrators. Nurse administrators must assume responsibility for disseminating information about the Nursing Minimum Data Set to their staff members and for encouraging the collection of standardized data. Use of the Nursing Minimum Data Set will test its applicability and provide information necessary for modification.

Although data sets must be developed and implemented rapidly, this does not negate the need for continued research in relation to patient outcomes responsive to nursing interventions. The use of patient outcomes as indicators of the quality of nursing care has a long history in nursing research. In the 1960s, Aydelotte (1962) examined behavioral and physical characteristics of patients as outcomes of nursing care. Since that time, patient outcomes have been used as a measure of nursing effectiveness in numerous studies (Heater, Becker, & Olson, 1988; Lang & Clinton, 1984; Marek, 1989; Peters, 1989; Taylor & Haussmann, 1988; Waltz & Strickland, 1989). A major nursing initiative on outcomes research was initiated by the National Center for Nursing Research (NCNR) in May of 1990 when it called together an expert planning group to discuss strategies for NCNR concerning patient outcomes and nursing research. This group coined the term *nurse-sensitive outcomes,* meaning those patient outcomes that are sensitive to nursing intervention. A follow-up state-of-the-science of nurse-sensitive patient outcomes research was held in the fall of 1991. The Center's efforts parallel an effort supported by the Agency for Health Care Policy and Research to develop a research agenda for outcomes and effectiveness research. In April 1991 a congressionally mandated conference to develop agendas for future research in 10 different areas of outcomes and effectiveness research was coordinated by the Foundation for Health Services Research. Despite the emphasis on patient outcomes in nursing research, a number of issues must be addressed to make findings more applicable for effectiveness research.

More rigor needs to be applied in the development of methodology and instrumentation for outcome measurement (Lang & Clinton,1984; Waltz & Strickland, 1989). In particular, stricter attention needs to be paid to the use of measurement principles in the development of outcome measures (Waltz & Strickland, 1989). The reliability and validity of instruments need to be reported consistently, and continued reliability and validity testing needs to be done with different populations and in different settings (Lang & Clinton, 1984). Continued testing of outcome methodology and instruments requires that available tools be applied to outcome research. Currently, repeated use of available instrumentation is less common than is the development of new measures. As an example, one of the early tools to be developed (Majesky, Brester, & Nishio, 1978) has received little use in outcomes research. This tool used physiologic factors and degree of self-care as outcome measures, but whether these factors are the most important outcomes can be determined only by repeated use. The tendency to develop new tools rather then to test available ones makes it difficult to develop valid, reliable tools and to determine significant nurse-sensitive outcomes, especially when samples used in nursing outcome research are not generally large. Greater use of meta-analysis, such as that by Heater and colleagues (1988), can offset some of the problems with sample size, but efforts need to be directed toward obtaining larger samples through the use of multiple sites and populations. The development of multiple sites will require greater collaboration between nurse administrators and researchers and a willingness to share information among nurse administrators.

Conceptual frameworks for the development of outcome criteria need to be developed to support outcome research in nursing. Reviews of current nursing research that uses outcome criteria highlight the fact that conceptual frameworks seldom are used to support the identification of outcome variables (Lang & Clinton, 1984; Waltz & Strickland, 1989).

Outcome research needs to be applied in all settings and with all populations. Much of the current work relates to hospitalized patients, despite the fact that nursing is the major health care provider in nursing homes and community settings. More outcome research also needs to be done with the gerontology and pediatric patient; the majority of studies to date have been done with young and midlife adult populations.

Linkages between structure and outcome and process and outcome need further study. Currently, there is limited research showing a causal link between nursing interventions and patient outcomes (Marek, 1989; Waltz & Strickland, 1989). In addition, Waltz and Strickland (1989) found that studies examining these relationships often do not differentiate process and outcome variables and in fact may use the same tool to make both variables operational.

Outcome research would benefit from closer collaboration between researchers and practitioners, particularly those responsible for quality assurance programs. Practitioners can identify issues that may not be readily apparent to researchers (Lang & Clinton, 1984), they can support outcome research in their settings, and perhaps most important, they can facilitate the use of outcome measures if they become committed to them through participation in the research process.

CONCLUSION

Outcomes have proved difficult to measure because they are an "immensely complex construct" (Lohr, 1988, p. 38). However, the mandate for health professionals is clear. If nursing is unable or unwilling to delineate expected outcomes and the methodology for measuring them, there is a very real danger that effectiveness research will not include nurse-sensitive outcomes or that such outcomes will be developed by those who are not nurses. Nursing must take advantage of this great opportunity to demonstrate its contributions to health care.

REFERENCES

Aiken L. (1988). Assuring the delivery of quality patient care. In *Nursing resources and the delivery of patient care* (NIH Publication No. 89-3008, pp. 3-10). Washington, DC: U.S. Government Printing Office.

Agency for Health Care Policy and Research (1990, February). *AHCPR program note: Nursing advisory panel for guideline development: Summary*, (DHHS). Washington, DC: U.S. Government Printing Office.

Agency for Health Care Policy and Research (1990, August). *AHCPR program note: Clinical guideline development* (DHHS), p. 2. Washington, DC: U.S. Government Printing Office.

Agency for Health Care Policy and Research (1990, September). *AHCPR: Purpose and programs* (DHHS). Washington, DC: U.S. Government Printing Office.

American Nurses' Association. (April 30–May 1, 1990). *Summary of action (minutes) Congress of Nursing Practice steering committee on databases to support clinical nursing practice*. Kansas City, MO: Author.

American Nurses' Association. (1990, October). ANA, new agency launch nursing standards project. *The American Nurse*, p. 11.

Aydelotte, M. (1962). The use of patient welfare as a criterion measure. *Nursing Research*, *11*(1), 10-14.

Ellwood, P. M. (1988). Shattuck lecture—Outcomes management a technology of patient experience. *New England Journal of Medicine, 318*, 1549-1556.

Grace, H. (1990). Can health care costs be contained? *Nursing and Health Care, 11*(3), 125-130.

Greenfield, S. (1990). What's the next step for outcomes assessment? *The Internist, 31*(1), 6-8, 10.

Heater, B. S., Becker, A. M., & Olson, R. K. (1988). Nursing interventions and patient outcomes: A meta-analysis of studies. *Nursing Research, 37,* 303-307.

Joint Commission on Accreditation of Healthcare Organizations. (1989). Clinical indicators for initial testing. (Set No. 2, Oncology patients, trauma patients, cardiovascular patients). Chicago: Author.

Joint Commission on Accreditation of Healthcare Organizations. (1990). Clinical indicators recommended for consideration in the monitoring and evaluation process. (Set No. 1, Obstetrics patients, anesthesia patients). Chicago: Author.

Lang, N. M., & Clinton, J. F. (1984). Assessment of quality of nursing care. In H. H. Werley & J. J. Fitzpatrick (Eds.), *Annual review of nursing research* (Vol. 2, pp. 135-163). New York: Springer.

Lohr, K. N. (1988). Outcome measurement: Concepts and questions. *Inquiry, 25*(1), 37-50.

Madden, D. L. (1990). Health groups, payers develop own "outcomes" programs. *The Internist, 31*(1), 8.

Majesky, S. J., Brester, M. H., & Nishio, K. T. (1978). Development of a research tool: Patient indicators of nursing care. *Nursing Research, 27,* 365-371.

Marek, K. D. (1989). Outcome measurement in nursing. *Journal of Nursing Quality Assurance, 4*(1), 1-9.

McCloskey, J. C., Bulechek, G. M., Cohen, M. Z., Craft, M. J., Crossley, J. D., Denehy, J. A., Glick, O. J., Kruckeberg, T., Maas, M., Prophet, C. M. & Tripp-Reimer, T. (1990). Classification of nursing interventions. *Journal of Professional Nursing, 6*(3), 151-157.

O'Connor, K. S. (1990). *Effectiveness and outcomes of health care services: Implications for nursing: Final report.* Kansas City, MO: American Nurses' Association.

O'Leary, D. (1987). The Joint Commission looks to the future [Editorial]. *JAMA, 258,* 951-952.

Peters, D. A. (1989). An overview of current research relating to long-term outcomes. *Nursing & Health Care, 10*(3), 133-136.

Roper, W. L. (1990). Seeking effectiveness in health care: The federal perspective. *The Internist, 31*(1), 9-10.

Roper, W. L., Winkenwerder, W., Hackbarth, G. M., & Krakauer, H. (1988). Effectiveness in health care and initiative to evaluate and improve medical practice. *New England Journal of Medicine, 319,* 1197-1202.

Simpson, R. L. (1991). Adopting a nursing minimum data set. *Nursing Management, 22*(2), 20-21.

Tarlov, A. R., Ware, J. E., Greenfield, S., Nelson, E. C., Perrin, E., & Zubkoff, M. (1989). The medical outcomes study: An application of methods for monitoring the results of medical care. *JAMA, 262,* 925-930.

Taylor, A. G., & Haussmann, G. M. (1988). Meaning and measurement of quality nursing care. *Applied Nursing Research, 1*(2), 84-88.

Waltz, C. F., & Strickland, O. L. (1989). Issues and imperatives in instrumentation in nursing research. In I. L. Abraham, D. M. Nadzam, & J. J. Fitzpatrick (Eds.), *Statistics and quantitative methods in nursing* (pp. 202-214). Philadelphia: Saunders.

Washington Focus. (1988). OBRA message is clear: Quality or bust. *Nursing & Health Care, 9*(3), 123-124.

Werley, H. H., & Lang, N. M. (1988). *Identification of the Nursing Minimum Data Set.* New York: Springer.

Wiltse, B. (1990, June 17). *Redefining quality for the 90's: JCAHO Agenda for Change.* Paper presented at the national meeting of the American Nurses' Association, Boston.

Wyszewianski, L. (1988). Quality of care: Past achievements and future challenges. *Inquiry, 25*(1), 25-36.

SECTION TWO

Applications for Quality

Issues related to the development and implementation of quality assurance and quality improvement programs are discussed in this section in relation to specific settings and programs. Current endeavors in program development and the strengths and weaknesses of various programs, as well as problems that have hindered the development of strong quality assurance programs, are discussed in these chapters.

The chapter by Reiley shows how some of the external forces described in previous chapters have generated a renewed interest in quality. The application to health care of five quality approaches used in industry is presented, and current models used for nursing quality assurance programs are discussed. In the following chapter, Zander provides a model that links process, structure, and outcome with the components of primary nursing, managed care, and case management delivery models. The model developed at the New England Medical Center is described and illustrated in relation to Zander's model. The concept of total quality management is outlined in the next chapter, and the implementation of this concept at the University of Michigan Medical Center is described by Marszalek-Gaucher.

The last two chapters discuss aspects of quality assurance specific to the community setting and to nursing homes. A discussion of current community accreditation programs, their requirements, and projected future is provided by Rooney. The multiple issues, including economic and policy issues, that face the nursing home industry are discussed by Harrington. The author uses the components of structure, process, and outcome to describe the current situation in nursing home care and to suggest change to achieve the preferred environment.

Each chapter provides information useful for nurse administrators in whatever type of organization they work. As lengths of stay in acute care facilities decrease, the need to provide continuity of care makes more apparent the necessity of understanding issues and problems that face related health care organizations.

CHAPTER 6

Quality Assurance Programs

Peggy Reiley

Quality assurance programs have suffered because of problems in defining and measuring quality. The five approaches used by Garvin to define quality are applicable to health care settings and can, in fact, provide a broader perspective of quality, as discussed in this chapter. Issues related to quality assurance programs have led to a number of strategies, such as unit-based quality assurance, concurrent monitoring, and interdisciplinary programs designed to resolve current problems. Attention also must be given to the collection and storage of data and the development of an organization-wide emphasis on quality. These aspects of quality assurance programs are discussed in this chapter.

The field of quality assurance and quality assessment is as old as modern nursing. In 1855 Florence Nightingale dramatically called attention to the abysmal conditions of the military hospitals during the Crimean War. When she first arrived in Crimea, she was appalled by the existing conditions. The barracks of the hospital were infested with rats and fleas. The surroundings were filth-laden. Initially however, her criticisms received little attention. She was, after all, only a nurse and a woman. Not easily discouraged, she began to collect data on hospital casualties. She faced the challenge not only of turning the data into information but also of making such a clear presentation of the data that

Beth Israel Hospital Boston, MA 02215.

Series on Nursing Administration — Volume III, 1992

action would have to be taken. With the help of William Farr, a pioneer in the use of graphic techniques, she created bar graphs to dramatically display the death rates of soldiers from contagious diseases. Her data provided the powerful force needed for change to occur. Within 5 months the death rate from contagious disease was one ninth of what it was earlier (Wadsworth, Stephens, & Godfrey, 1986). This was truly an effective quality assurance program.

Florence Nightingale also was the first to write about standards of nursing practice. In her book *Notes on Nursing* she proposed standards for noise control, consistency of food, when food should be served, type of bed mattress to be used, position of the bed in relation to the window, cleanliness and airiness of the room, and personal cleanliness (Maibusch, 1984).

The modern era of quality assurance began in 1966. It was during this time that the American Nurses' Association created divisions for the purpose of developing standards of nursing care. These standards were to be utilized in the development of quality assurance programs (Smeltzer, 1988). These early programs were developed primarily by monitoring care and determining its conformance with standards of practice. The medical record was used as a primary data source for the monitoring activities.

PROBLEMS IN THE DEVELOPMENT OF QUALITY ASSURANCE

Although the early work was exciting and the field of quality assurance continued to grow and expand in nursing, it did not keep pace with other areas of nursing, such as research. Quality assurance in nursing, like quality assurance in medicine, has struggled with a number of problems. Chief among these is that quality has been difficult to measure. There are a number of reasons why measurement has proved difficult.

One reason is that patients, even though they may have the same medical diagnosis, may have varying levels of health related problems. In addition, there is no clear agreement on what our product should be. In industry the development of standards and the measurement of quality seem rather simple. In health care, this is not as easy. Often there are either no standards or a lack of agreement about which standards should be used to evaluate quality.

Another reason that quality has been difficult to measure is the autonomy of professionals and the hesitation to "criticize" each other. Nursing professionals have found it difficult to give each other negative feedback about the quality of nursing care that patients receive. Quality assurance programs have little hope for effectiveness if professionals are not willing to critique or to be critiqued. The knowledge base of nursing science has been ambiguous, which has contributed to problems in the measurement of nursing care quality. As our knowledge base expands, we should be able to better measure the quality of nursing care.

Finally, and perhaps most important, it has been difficult to develop meaningful measures of quality because quality has not been viewed as an urgent issue until recently. Health care professionals have not shown the same interest in quality as they have in other aspects of practice. The general attitude of health care providers has been that the quality of care patients receive is good, even though inadequately measured. It is primarily because of external forces that health care providers now have an increased interest in measuring the quality of health care.

The Impact of External Forces on Quality

Concerns about quality have increased as a result of cost containment efforts, particularly the introduction of prospective payment. Consumers and regulators are questioning the effect that cost containment has on the quality of health care services.

Prospective payment. Chief among the external forces is a fear that the prospective payment system (DRGs) will have a negative impact on the quality of care. When Congress passed the Social Security Amendments of 1983 (Public Law 98-21), the traditional cost-based method of reimbursement for Medicare patients was changed to a prospective payment system and completely changed the incentives by which hospitals operate. In the old cost-based system of reimbursement there were few incentives to control costs (Gutterman & Dobson, 1986), because higher costs meant higher rates of reimbursement. In the new prospective payment system there are clear incentives to control costs and to provide care at the lowest possible cost. Many consumers, regulators, and health care providers are concerned that lower-cost care also may mean lower-quality care.

In analyzing the economic incentives inherent in prospective payment, it is possible to postulate that the quality of care may be adversely affected; it also is possible to postulate that the quality of care may be positively affected. For example, one of the economic incentives operative in prospective payment is to reduce the length of hospital stay. This change could negatively affect the quality of care if patients are discharged from the hospital too quickly or before they or their families are able to properly care for them at home. If this were to occur with any frequency, there could be an increase in the posthospitalization death rate or patients might be readmitted to the hospital sicker and more debilitated.

On the other hand, a reduced length of stay may positively affect the quality of care if the psychologic state of the patient is enhanced by not being in the "sick role" for a prolonged period of time. In addition, with reduced lengths of stay, patients will have a decreased risk of hospital-acquired diseases, such as urinary tract infections and complications from test procedures. The patient's ability to maintain independence in function also may be promoted with a decreased length of stay. Elderly patients in particular may sustain functional decline with prolonged hospitalization. Early discharge may prevent the occurrence of these complications.

Another economic condition inherent in prospective payment is the incentive to decrease the use of ancillary services. Again, the results can have positive or negative effects on the quality of care. Quality will be enhanced if needless tests or procedures are abolished. If, however, needed tests or procedures are withheld to reduce costs, then the quality of care will be diminished. An example is the preventive testing that is so necessary for the early detection of disease. If hospitals curtail routine Papanicolaou's testing and treat only the disease for which the patient is hospitalized, early stages of uterine disease may be missed, with subsequent disastrous effects on the health status of women.

There also is the incentive for hospitals to increase specialization, particularly among those DRGs that are not profitable. Increased specialization can enhance the quality of care. Several studies have shown that high case volume is associated with lower morbidity and mortality (Luft & Hunt, 1986; Riley & Lubitz, 1985). Specialization also can have a negative impact on the quality of care if hospitals choose to specialize only in those cases that are highly profitable and ignore those that are unprofitable. Access to care would be limited if this were to occur.

A final incentive of the prospective payment system is for hospitals to do a more thorough assessment of the costs and benefits of various technologies. This could enhance quality if hospitals choose to focus on prevention and not only on expensive after-the-fact technologies. It also could diminish quality if access to high-cost intensive care units is limited or, if lifesaving, although costly, technologies are not adopted.

It is clear that this reimbursement system has affected not only Medicare patients but virtually all hospitalized patients. The length of stay fell by almost 1 day in 1984 (Gutterman & Dobson, 1986). Hospitals are responding to the current economic incentives. This dramatic response to these financial incentives has renewed interest in quality assessment and measurement.

Increased consumerism. Another reason that quality has emerged as the issue of the nineties is the increased consumer interest and demand for quality health care services. In the past, medical professionals were, for the most part, immune from questions regarding their professional judgment, and patients by and large passively allowed whatever treatments their physician deemed necessary. Today these relationships are changing, and consumers are demanding that hospitals and health care professionals be accountable for the quality of care delivered. The number of malpractice claims initiated against physicians is one indicator that the public is indeed scrutinizing the quality of medical care.

One attempt to assist consumers evaluate the quality of medical care was the government's publication of a list of 2300 hospitals that had unusually high or low death or utilization rates. The list was first developed with use of 1984 Medicare claims data from approximately 11 million Medicare patients. Overall mortality rates were predicted by means of national norms, which were adjusted for 90 variables such as age, race, and sex. The hospitals' actual mortality rates were then compared with national norms. The release of this information initiated angry protests from hospitals, largely because the data were thought to be spurious, with no adjustments for the severity of illness. Consumers, however, praised the Health Care Financing Administration for these efforts (*American Medical News,* 1986), thereby contributing to the renewed interest in quality.

Increased interest from regulators. In 1965, with the enactment of Medicare and Medicaid, the government became the largest purchaser of health care services. The passing of this momentous piece of legislation was not without formidable foes, chief among them the American Medical Association. To placate the American Medical Association the government made a number of concessions, one being that it would not interfere with the autonomy of the medical profession. Thus the regulation of physician practice was not part of the early Medicare program.

It is unrealistic to expect the government to have no voice in how services are delivered when health care costs exceed 12% of our gross national product and government bears much of this cost. One of the first government-directed regulatory bodies, the Professional Standards Review Organization (PSRO), was established in 1972. PSRO was to oversee utilization of Medicare services, as well as to assess the quality of care. The reality is, however, that the PSRO did little in quality assessment.

With the passing of the Tax Equity and Fiscal Responsibility Act of 1982, the need for greater regulation of quality of care was recognized. Peer review organizations were established to take over the function of the PSRO but with greater emphasis on assessment of quality. Thus an increased emphasis on the measurement and assessment of quality grew out of regulatory efforts. All these factors have forced the issue of quality to the forefront of health care concerns but have not resolved problems associated with the evaluation of quality.

DEFINING QUALITY

Before quality can be measured or assessed, it must be defined. Quality is a construct that, like freedom or liberty, cannot be measured directly. To be measured, quality must be defined operationally. Perhaps one of the reasons health care providers have trouble measuring quality is the tendency to define it too narrowly, either by conformance to standards of the Joint Commission for the Accreditation of Healthcare Organizations or by standards of regulatory agencies.

Garvin (1988) has defined quality from an industrial perspective. He suggests five approaches for defining quality and discusses the advantages and disadvantages of each approach. These approaches may be useful to define the quality of care that patients receive.

The first approach for defining quality is the transcendent view. This approach is similar to Plato's discussion of beauty, in that quality, like beauty, can be understood only after continuous exposure to it. Once its meaning is exposed and understood, quality is absolute and universally recognized. We have all heard colleagues speak of quality as something that is hard to define but "you know it when you see it." The problem with this approach is that quality remains elusive and perhaps identifiable to only a few. Objective measures of quality cannot be derived from definitions of quality based on this approach.

The second approach provides a product-based definition of quality. By means of this definition, quality is both measurable and precise. For example, it might be the percentage of wool in a skirt or the amount of butterfat in ice cream. From a health care perspective, it might be the number of private rooms or the type of food served. The advantage of a product-based definition is that quality becomes more measurable. There also are a number of disadvantages with the use of a product-based definition. One is that high quality almost always means higher costs. Another is that a correlation between quality and the product attributes does not always exist. Finally, this definition of quality does not take consumer preferences into account. For example, not all patients prefer private rooms or the same type of food.

A third approach is the user-based definition of quality. With this approach, quality, like beauty, is in the eyes of the beholder. Thus quality is that which satisfies the majority of consumers. Application of this approach in health care would require careful consideration of patient satisfaction data. The advantage of a user-based definition is that it takes consumer preferences into consideration. A disadvantage of such a definition is that consumer tastes differ, and to satisfy the majority may be difficult. Also, the preferences of the majority may not be synonymous with the highest quality. For example, acid rock may surpass classical music in sales, but few people would argue that the quality of acid rock music is truly superior. In health care there are many clinicians who argue that consumers are not informed enough to accurately assess the quality of health care and that the consumer's measures of quality may be very different from the medical standards of quality.

A fourth approach utilizes a manufacturing-based definition of quality. In this approach, quality is defined as "conformance to established standards." Such standards generally are established by experts in the field. Health care professionals have made extensive use of this approach with professional and organizational standards of practice. One advantage of this definition is that conformance with standards is a way to measure quality. Another advantage is that consumer interest is acknowledged inasmuch as nonconformance with standards implies an inferior product and possible consumer dissatisfaction. The disadvantage of this definition is that it is too internal. The link between nonconformance and consumer dissatisfaction is supposed but not proved. The standards developed may have nothing to do with quality from the perspective of the consumer. In health care, for example, care may be delivered that is technologically superior, the standards of care absolutely adhered to, and clinical excellence evident; if, however, it is delivered in an inhumane way, from the consumers' perspective the quality of care may be poor.

Garvin's final approach to quality creates a value-based definition. Here quality is defined in terms of costs. A quality product is one that produces conformance to standards at an acceptable cost. Thus if a product is overpriced, regardless of the inherent quality, it would not be considered high quality because of the excessive price. The prospective payment system could be thought of as an attempt to move to a more value-based definition of quality. Garvin states that despite the importance of this definition, it is difficult to blend the two concepts of excellence and worth, and what one obtains is a hybrid "affordable excellence."

Which of these definitions is most meaningful in health care? I would suggest that we discontinue our narrow definitions of quality and incorporate all these definitions into our quality assurance programs. The assessment of quality based on standards should be only one dimension to our assessment of quality. Health care providers need to incorporate user-based definitions, product-based definitions, and value-based definitions to accurately assess the quality of care.

CHANGES IN QUALITY ASSURANCE PROGRAMS

Quality assurance programs are in a state of flux because of changes in the external environment and the way in which quality is being defined. The remainder of this chapter provides an overview of the evolution taking place in quality assurance programs.

Unit-Based Quality Assurance

There have been a number of recent, positive advances in quality assurance programs; chief among them is the movement from a centralized to decentralized system, utilizing the unit-based approach. In the centralized approach to quality assurance, monitoring was conducted by individuals who were not actually delivering care to patients. This posed a number of problems. First of all, although the data generated from such centralized activities may be useful, it may be impossible for the individuals doing the monitoring to intervene with corrective action if they are

Unit-Based Quality Assurance Committee

Hospital-Wide Quality Assurance Nursing Committee

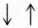

Interdisciplinary Quality Assurance Committee

FIG 6-1 A quality assurance committee structure.

not delivering the care (Beyerman, 1987). The ability of such programs to truly affect the quality of care is limited when staff members who provide care are not involved in the quality assurance process.

The unit-based approach to quality assurance addresses these issues. It is based on the idea that the individuals actually providing the care ought to be the ones monitoring the quality of that care. The personnel providing the care should determine which aspects of care are to be monitored and should develop plans for corrective action.

There are a number of advantages with a unit-based quality assurance system. The potential to actually improve the quality of care is enhanced because personnel delivering the care are involved in the process. When staff members decide which aspects of quality are meaningful to measure, the assessment of quality becomes alive and exciting. The data generated are useful, and consequently the staff is more willing to take corrective action on identified problems. This approach enhances the nurse's role and the image of nursing. Through the quality assurance process of collecting and analyzing data applicable to their unit, nurses learn what constitutes high-quality care and how their individual contributions affect health care quality (Formella & Schroeder, 1984).

There also are some potential drawbacks to the unit-based approach. The most important is that, because the focus is at the unit level, there may be little opportunity to share monitoring activities or plans for corrective action across units. This problem can be avoided if there is a mechanism built into the system to share such activities. A potential structure for sharing quality assurance activities is illustrated in Fig. 6-1. The basis of the model is the unit-based quality assurance committee. The responsibilities for this committee might include the following:

- Identifying practice issues for monitoring
- Coordinating and ensuring unit-based monitoring by incorporating clinical nurses
- Developing and implementing plans for corrective action
- Following-up on corrective action plan
- Reporting results of quality assurance activities to all unit staff members

The next level is the hospital-wide nursing quality assurance committee, which ideally should consist of a representative from each of the unit-based committees. This committee would be broader in scope, and its activities might include the following:

- Evaluating nursing department standards of care
- Determining the need for new standards
- Identifying and sharing practice issues to be monitored
- Sharing plans for corrective action
- Sharing all unit-based quality assurance activities

The final level is an interdisciplinary quality assurance committee. This committee should include the heads of all clinical services. The purpose of this committee is to share quality assurance activities of each discipline and to explore opportunities for interdisciplinary quality assurance activities.

An additional potential drawback to the unit-based model is the potential for bias as nurses evaluate the practice of peers on their own unit. Bias can be avoided by having well-defined, explicit criteria for the monitoring process. If quality assurance is approached from the positive aspect of an opportunity to improve practice rather than from the traditional problem-identification approach, nurses will be more likely to evaluate the practice of their peers objectively.

Quality Councils

Another interesting development in quality assurance programs is the use of quality councils. The "council" is a governing body that oversees the quality of care patients receive. Such councils might be population specific. For example, the cardiac council might include nurses from the coronary care unit, step-down unit, cardiac catheterization laboratory, surgical intensive care unit, operating room, home care, and cardiology clinic. The council would be responsible for developing standards and assessing and monitoring the quality of care that all cardiac patients receive.

This model has very exciting possibilities for truly affecting patient outcomes. Our traditional quality assurance programs have narrow boundaries if based just at the unit level. Because most patients move through various departments and units, it would seem reasonable that our quality assurance programs should do the same.

Ideally, councils are interdisciplinary in nature, with each discipline making a contribution to standards development, as well as monitoring activities. The focus of the interdisciplinary council is on the patient rather than on the provider. Focusing on the patient promotes the development of outcome standards as well as process standards.

Concurrent Monitoring

Most quality assurance activities of the past have involved retrospective intermittent chart reviews that primarily looked at the application of the nursing process. That is, a number of charts were audited on a retrospective, intermittent basis, and the primary focus was on the presence or absence of documentation.

There are a number of problems with this approach. The presence of documentation serves as a proxy for quality and does not really ensure the presence of quality. The retrospective system can do little to actually improve the quality of care of current patients, because the assessment of quality is after the fact. Finally, intermittent assessment of quality does little to improve practice inasmuch as a continuous feedback loop is not possible when quality is monitored intermittently.

The change to ongoing, continuous monitoring of primary indicators of care has been brought about largely through requirements of the Joint Commission (1989, p. 75). The Joint Commission allows each institution to determine the primary indicators of care used in monitoring but suggests that institutions look at high volume, high risk, or problem cases in developing monitors.

High-volume cases are easy for nursing services to identify. One way to assess high-volume cases is to look at hospital utilization data. If such an analysis shows that the largest number of medical patients are admitted for cardiac problems, it is logical to monitor the care of the cardiac patient. Another way of assessing high volume is to determine those nursing activities that are performed frequently regardless of case type. Patient teaching and discharge planning are two nursing functions that are consistently provided to all patients and therefore would be considered high volume.

Aspects of care in which there is high risk to the patient also should be monitored, for example, patient falls, medication errors, and self-extubation in the critical care areas. Although the volume of these particular cases may not be high, the potential for injury to the patient is so great that monitoring becomes essential. A final component that must be monitored is those aspects of care in which problems either have been identified or are suspected. These problems may derive from a failure to adhere to standards or protocols or from the failure to achieve specified patient outcomes.

Standards of care are used as guidelines for the development of monitors. As such, standards of care are less likely to be ignored and more likely to be applied to current practice. The use of standards in the evaluation of care will have a positive effect on the assurance of quality.

Interdisciplinary Quality Assurance

One of the results of the prospective payment reimbursement system created by the Tax Equity and Fiscal Responsibility Act (TEFRA) is that hospitalized patients today are far sicker and in need of more complex care. The increased complexity of care often requires the services of multiple health care professionals, but no one discipline is totally responsible for patient outcomes. An evaluation of total patient care therefore should demonstrate the accountabilities, deficiencies, and achievements of all health care team members (Mosleth, 1984).

For a number of years the Joint Commission has recognized that the ultimate quality of patient care depends on a number of disciplines and has required that specialty units conduct multidisciplinary quality assurance activities. There is a need to go further and to develop interdisciplinary quality assurance activities in all patient care areas. There is very little in the literature regarding interdisciplinary quality assurance. An excellent study (Knaus, Draper, Wagner, Zimmerman, 1968) looked at the Health Care Financing Administration outcome data to determine factors that account for poor or good outcomes of care in intensive care units. After adjusting for severity of illness, the authors looked at both high and low outliers to determine variables that might account for such outcomes. They found the most important variable to be the relationship of the medical and nursing staffs in regard to their ability to collaborate effectively.

More studies and more collaborative efforts in quality assurance are needed for health professions. There is no doubt of the agreement among all disciplines that the unifying goal is high-quality patient care. This goal might be better achieved through collaborative action in quality assurance.

Patient Satisfaction

The measurement of patient satisfaction with the quality of care received has gained increased interest over the past several years for a number of reasons. One is the rise in consumerism discussed earlier. Another is that health care providers have come to realize that client satisfaction may be the key to institutional survival in the increasingly competitive health care market (Elbeck, 1987).

Members of the Technical Assistance Research Programs (Petersen, 1988) attempted to calculate the cost to the hospital of one dissatisfied patient and projected the following consequences:

- One dissatisfied consumer will inform 10 friends.
- Of those 10, one is considering using the facility.
- One of five would have chosen the facility.
- One of three who hears the dissatisfied friend will not choose the facility.

The cost of these consequences can be calculated as follows:

$(10 \times 0.1 \times 0.2 \times 0.33) \times \$5000$ (estimated average revenue per patient) $= \$330$ (cost of each dissatisfied patient)

Patient satisfaction is an outcome measured from the perspective of the patient. Measuring patient satisfaction with nursing care permits a broader definition of quality. It is critical to obtain measures of patient satisfaction that yield reliable data regarding the patient's perception of nursing care. One such instrument is the Patient Satisfaction Instrument (Bader, 1988). It consists of 25 items with three subscales. The first subscale, the professional-technical, measures the patient's perception of the nurse's knowledge of nursing, the physical care received, and the implementation of the medical plan of care. The second subscale addresses patient teaching and measures the adequacy of information exchange between the nurse and the patient. The third subscale is trust, which measures the nurse's sensitivity and listening skills from the patient's perspective.

Automation of Data Sources

In the past, the patient record was the primary data source used for quality assurance studies in nursing. Although useful, this data source has its limitations. One is that it may not accurately reflect the quality of care that patients receive. Another limitation is that it is often time-consuming to retrieve data from the medical record. For these reasons other data sources such as incident reports, direct observation, and patient interview have been explored for quality assurance studies. An exciting development is the use of the computer to store and analyze data. The outcome data of the Health Care Financing Administration is an example of how large numbers of cases can be analyzed with use of a computer. Nursing is beginning to develop data bases that will assist in the evaluation of patient care. One potential source of quality assurance data that is largely untapped is the patient classification systems used in most hospitals. Primarily designed to capture information on nursing resource utilization for budgetary and staffing purposes, most patient classification systems also provide a source of excellent clinical information. The challenge for nursing is to determine how this clinical information can be used for quality assurance purposes.

Computerization of quality assurance data also may be useful for more thorough data analyses, as well as for trending purposes. There are a number of data base, spreadsheet, and statistical packages available that can be used for these analyses. Knowledge of software packages and their use is critical for any nurse involved in quality assurance.

Medicus has developed a personal computer–based quality assurance software package. Information is collected primarily from an audit of nursing records and then sent to a central computer for analysis. The type of data collected is primarily that regarding compliance with nursing standards. The system is used by a number of institutions, and it is therefore possible to make institutional comparisons regarding care received (Greer & Hexum, 1987).

As health care organizations move into the world of automation, the potential for obtaining and analyzing large amounts of data for quality assurance purposes will expand. As more institutions move to automated nursing assessments, care plans, and documentation, it will be possible to obtain valuable patient information in less time than with traditional record reviews.

Performance

One of the basic ways of ensuring the quality of patient care is to ensure that the personnel caring for patients are competent, capable, and caring. Ensuring competence requires the development of structure and process standards in four areas: entry requirements, performance expectations, continuing education, and performance appraisal (Porter, 1988).

Licensure is the most basic entry requirement. Licensure assures the institution that the individual has completed a basic nursing curriculum and has mastered the course content well enough to pass the licensure examination. An institution may set other entry requirements in addition to the requirement of licensure. For example, an institution may elect to hire only nurses with a baccalaureate degree. Although these structure requirements are only indicators of an individual provider's competence, they can be a useful screening tool.

Setting performance expectations usually is accomplished through a well-developed job description. Many institutions also have orientation programs that specify the level of competency expected at the completion of the program. Generic expectations based on uniform nursing functions, such as teaching or using the nursing process, also set performance standards.

Continuing education is critical to keep staff members updated and informed about practice. Continuing education in its most basic form should assist in maintaining competence and ideally should assist in professional growth and development. Continuing education activities should, in part, be built around the results of quality assurance findings. For example, if through quality assurance monitoring it is found that nurses are not teaching patients in the expected manner, a continuing education program on patient education would be appropriate.

Performance appraisal is another method of ensuring quality. Performance appraisals give the clinician being appraised, as well as the manager and peers, the opportunity to discuss individual strengths and weaknesses in meeting performance standards. They provide the opportunity to explore ways to assist the individual nurse to grow and to develop as a professional, as well as to evaluate performance. The quality of care that patients receive ultimately depends on the competency of those delivering the care. That is why performance standards and appraisal are critical elements of the quality assurance process.

A New View of Quality

One of the more recent and profound changes in quality assurance programs is a movement toward hospital-wide quality control. This broader view of quality stems from industrial application of a total quality concept. Sullivan (1986) describes total quality as a system "to economically produce goods or service which satisfy customers' requirements" (p. 77).

Many health care institutions have recently become interested in this strategic approach to quality, which differs from the traditional approach in a number of ways. It recognizes that quality assurance and control are everybody's business, not just those given the specific job function of ensuring quality; it also encourages a top level commitment to quality that often is lacking in the more traditional setting. In addition, it stimulates an increased awareness of consumers and their views of the quality of care.

Why have many hospitals suddenly become interested in the more strategic approach to quality? The answer quite simply is survival. Administrators have looked at industry and found that the development of a total quality program could give them a significant competitive advantage. From a nursing perspective, this change in focus has exciting possibilities. When quality is everybody's job—dietary personnel, housekeepers, laboratory technicians—the potential for collaboration to solve systems problems and to improve patient care is endless.

CONCLUSION

The field of quality assurance, after years of little progress, is now undergoing dramatic changes based on a renewed interest in quality—among providers, consumers, and regulators. All indications are that quality will be better assessed and measured in the future. Consumers may look at quality data to determine which institutions they will choose. Payers of health care services also may use quality indicators to determine whether to pay for a service.

The challenge for nursing is to develop reliable and valid measures to assess the quality of nursing care and to develop strategies to improve the nursing care quality. Last, nurses also need to develop more research-based quality assurance studies and to share their findings with their colleagues.

REFERENCES

American Medical News, March 21, 1986.

Bader, M. M. (1988). Nursing care behaviors that predict patient satisfaction. *Journal of Nursing Quality Assurance*, 2(3), 11-17.

Beyerman, K. (1987). Developing a unit-based nursing quality assurance program: From concept to practice. *Journal of Nursing Quality Assurance*, 2(1), 1-11.

Elbeck, M. (1987). An approach to client satisfaction measurement as an attribute of health service quality. *Health Care Management Review, 12,*(3), 47-52.

Formella, N. M., & Schroeder, P. S. (1984). The unit-based system. In P. S. Schoeder & R. M. Maibusch (Eds.). *Nursing quality assurance: A unit-based approach*. Rockville, MD: Aspen.

Garvin, D. A. (1988). *Managing quality*. New York: Macmillan.

Greer, J., & Hexum, J. (1987). Dimensions of computerized quality assurance systems. *Journal of Nursing Quality Assurance, 1*(4), 9-14.

Gutterman, S., & Dobson, A. (1986). Impact of the Medicare prospective payment system for hospitals. *Health Care Financing Review, 7*(1), 97-114.

Joint Commission on Accreditation of Hospitals: (1989). *Monitoring and evaluation of the quality and appropriateness of care*. Chicago: Author.

Knaus, W., Draper, E., Wagner, D., & Zimmerman, Y. (1968). An evaluation of outcomes from intensive care in major medical centers. *Annals of Internal Medicine, 104,* 410-418.

Luft, H. S., & Hunt, S. (1986). Evaluating individual hospital quality through outcome statistics. *Journal of the American Medical Association, 255,* 2780-2784.

Maibusch, R. M. (1984). Evolution of quality assurance for nursing in hospitals. In P. S. Schroeder & R. M. Maibusch (Eds.). *Nursing quality assurance: A unit-based approach*. Rockville, MD: Aspen.

Mosleth, R. R. (1984). A practical guide to multi-disciplinary auditing. In P. S. Schroeder & R. M. Maibusch (Eds.). *Nursing quality assurance: A unit-based approach*. Rockville, MD: Aspen.

Petersen, M. B. H. (1988). Measuring patient satisfaction: Collecting useful data. *Journal of Nursing Quality Assurance, 2*(3), 25-35.

Porter, A. L. (1988). Assuring quality through staff nurse performance. *Nursing Clinics of North America, 23,* 649-655.

Riley, G., & Lubitz, J. (1985). Outcomes of surgery among the Medicare aged: Surgical volume and mortality. *Health Care Financing Review, 6,* 37-41.

Smeltzer, C. H. (1988). Evaluating a successful quality assurance program: The process. *Journal of Nursing Quality Assurance, 2*(4), 1-10.

Sullivan, L. P. (1986, May). The seven stages in company-wide quality control. *Quality Progress*, pp. 77-83.

Wadsworth, H. M., Stephens, K. S., & Godfrey, B. A. (1986). *Modern methods for quality control and improvement*. New York: John Wiley & Sons.

CHAPTER 7

Nursing Care Delivery Methods and Quality

Karen Zander

Until the advent of managed care and nursing case management as clinical systems to improve the way clinicians organize and process their work, nursing care delivery methods were considered the key mechanism to ensure quality. Methods such as functional or primary nursing, however, are relatively untested and, at best, are only the structural component of a complicated formula for producing quality processes and outcomes. This chapter deals with major considerations in the areas of work design, role, and feedback. Systems that provide the maximal predictability and consistency of quality clinical outcome are suggested.

The complex relationship between nursing care delivery methods and the quality of nursing care provided is essentially underdeveloped and underresearched. By necessity, nursing care delivery methods should be fluid and adaptive to the ever-changing clinical needs of the patient population. Yet too often, tradition, convenience (personal or geographic), and crisis determine the way patients' needs are matched to nursing resources. The quality of that match is subjectively determined by multiple players. Although everyone would agree that standards of quality should *drive* delivery methods, quality usually is the dependent variable—the final overlay rather than the first consideration. This

The Center for Nursing Care Management, Inc., 6 Pleasant Street, South Natick, MA 01760.

Series on Nursing Administration—Volume III, 1992

chapter explores the multidimensional equation between delivery methods and quality. Examples from preprimary nursing, primary nursing, mixed methods, managed care, and case management will be compared as models that combine various components of care delivery important to patients, nurses, and other key groups.

GENERAL CONSIDERATIONS

For quality to be totally integrated into the minds and hearts and behavior of every member of a nursing staff, there must be a consensual definition of quality, a unit milieu that is conducive to quality, and a clear cause-and-effect relationship between actions and their results. Quality does not necessarily mean meeting all needs of each patient, but it does mean responding to those needs that are important to a patient's overall sense of security and physical stability. A balance must be struck between ideal and possible, as well as between needs and the available resources to meet those needs.

There may be situations in which quality is high although individual staff nurse accountability is low. A busy day-surgery area may have functional nursing but, because the care is so regimented, may achieve consistent quality outcomes. There also may be situations in which roles are well developed and quite sophisticated but in which quality is not necessarily high. Of course there always are cases in which quality is high by clinician standards but not perceived that way by patients!

Contrary to popular belief, the equation between a given delivery method and quality is not linear and cannot be noted as X delivery method equals mega quality; Y delivery method equals minus quality. Nursing care will never be quite that simplistic! Some general considerations, however, which are at the root of all discussions about care delivery methods and quality, follow.

1. There are very few "pure" care delivery methods 24 hours a day. This inconsistency is due to varying personnel standards per shift. For example, the RN supply can range from a base of one charge RN per shift to one RN per patient. Needs for additional caregivers may be filled only by RNs or by LPNs, aides, medication technicians, corpsmen, or other personnel. Which category is responsible for which activities is dictated by law, policy, and in some cases, convenience. *To wed a care delivery method to specific mix of staff may be restrictive.* For instance, to say that in primary nursing there must be an all-RN staff is neither true nor realistic in many settings.

2. No matter what the delivery method, an incompetent caregiver cannot provide any degree of quality. A marginally skilled or undermotivated staff member, however, may become functional and reasonably attentive if surrounded by a staff that is highly supportive and productive.

3. There are very few homogeneous nursing staffs, either in educa-

tional preparation or in job category. Most nursing staffs represent a mix of formal and professional experience. Even if each staff member has a Bachelor of Science in Nursing (BSN) degree, each nurse may favor a different theoretic model and have a particular style of interaction.

4. It is not sameness of degree, background, or title that unites staff members in a care delivery model; it is the manager. There must be a "fit" between the care delivery method and the manager's skill, knowledge, value system, and style. Otherwise a given delivery method, no matter how intrinsically "good," will not work on that unit. Although many excuses will be given, the manager, rather than the delivery method, is the focal point of a staff's behavior.

5. In addition to excellent management, the basic design of the care delivery system must be a *pattern.* In other words, it must (a) be relatively simple, (b) be easy to replicate and transfer, (c) fit most situations, and (d) provide direction rapidly. For example, team nursing is a relatively simple pattern with clear rules, adaptable to whatever mix of personnel report to work on a given shift. Another pattern uses the principle of continuity first, acuity second, and geography third in the assignment of patients to RNs who have been off duty 1 day or more.

6. Each unit has a pattern, as well as some important historical, emotional, and practical reasons to justify that pattern. Changes in the pattern, however faulty the pattern may be, threaten the staff's sense of stability and well-being. This feeling often gets misinterpreted as a threat to quality care, which makes objective dialogue among staff members difficult at best.

7. Inpatient nursing is always a group activity by nature. No matter what the care delivery system, nurses need physical help during a shift to give care and to cover breaks. There is enormous interdependence among individuals for care delivery during each shift and for information exchange at shift report. In addition, mutual clinical consultation and emotional support are interpersonal activities that help the care delivery system function effectively. Finally, the way non-unit-based persons and departments (physicians, laundry, laboratories, and admitting) are organized has a major impact on the nursing care delivery system and its potential for quality.

8. In terms of learning and working style, nurses tend to be more oriented toward the auditory and visual than toward reading and writing. Therefore a care delivery method must be based on observing and listening cues, as well as clues to receive and transfer information. In other words, documentation and written standards of care will not drive the delivery method unless and until they are incorporated into the prevalent way that nurses assimilate and use knowledge. Thus change-of-shift reports provide a more powerful communication system than do recorded progress notes in the chart.

9. Nursing care delivery methods are shift-centered methods wherein

the time limits of the shift dictate the prioritization of the activities. For nurses also to be "patient centered"—that is, to pay attention to the individual patient's needs and timelines during the hospital course— requires a second level of thought and action beyond setting priorities. In stressful situations this second level often deteriorates. Ideally, the quality characteristic of patient-centeredness is achieved through the concept of continuity. One way in which care delivery models can be compared is by the degree of formal continuity achieved in both the plan of care and the execution of that plan by "continuous" caregivers.

10. Care delivery methods also can be compared by their ability to help patients reach quality-level physiologic, functional, and knowledge outcomes. These outcomes are resolutions of problems, such as "potential for extension of the disease process," "potential for complications related to treatment," "potential for complications unrelated to treatment," and "potential for complications of self-care" (Stetler & DeZell, 1987, pp. 26-32). These problems, as well as the interventions to resolve them, describe nursing's special contribution to quality toward which care delivery systems must be geared. Although it is commonly held that nurses are task-centered, it also must be understood that nurses are fundamentally outcome driven (Zander, 1988a). The formalization of this basic truth into care delivery methods has only recently been undertaken. As nurses understand their role in outcome management and consciously define and manage toward outcomes, better care delivery methods will evolve.

RESPONSIBILITY AND ACCOUNTABILITY

Care delivery methods, which depend on more than semantic analysis, can be differentiated in two fundamental ways: their locus of responsibility for task completion and, second, the assignment of accountability for the consequences of those tasks. Four methods traditionally used to organize the work group for purposes of delivering care are (1) functional nursing, (2) team nursing, (3) total patient care, and (4) mixed methods.

These terms identify who does what and who reports to whom. Each method must include a nursing care plan and may include provisions for continuity of caregivers. These methods may be used as part of accountability models, such as primary nursing, but usually are stand-alone methods, implemented for the completion of work each shift. Their focus is essentially on tasks and process. In the absence of primary nursing, accountability for the *results* of those tasks for every patient is held at the nurse-manager level.

Primary nursing, and the new modes of case management discussed later, are the only two methods that decentralize accountability for outcomes for specific patients to the staff nurse. A variety of care delivery methods may be used within a primary nursing system, as long as each patient has a primary nurse who is his or her caregiver whenever on duty and who sets systems in place to help each primary patient achieve realistic, individualized outcomes (see box on p. 91). Primary nursing is *not* synonymous with total patient care, although a primary nurse may give total patient care to his or her primary patients. Total patient care is a responsibility method that terminates at the end of each shift. Primary nursing is an accountability method that specifies caseloads of two to six patients (national range) for which an individual nurse is accountable for outcomes whether on or off duty.

There generally are seven ways — sometimes overlapping — in which primary nurses can be assigned to caseloads of patients: (1) automatic/assigned/negotiated, (2) paired with specific physician(s), (3) special needs or case types, (4) return admissions, (5) geographically grouped, (6) "adoption" (RN choice), and (7) random.

Practice standards can be maintained best by the use of No. 1, with combinations of Nos. 2 through 5. Otherwise, primary nursing becomes a system for motivated nurses and their fortunate patients rather than a standard of practice across the board. Basically, *there is no such thing as "modified" primary nursing — either the head nurse has decentralized accountability for individualized sets of outcomes to the staff or has kept that accountability.* On the other hand, there can be such a thing as modified total patient care or team nursing, depending on the shift and the resources.

There is a great deal of ambivalence among managers and staff nurses toward accountability. Not every staff nurse desires accountability, and not every manager knows how to make staff accountable. Most helpful to this discussion is Bergman's model of the preconditions leading to accountability: (1) ability (knowledge, skills, values), (2) responsibility, and (3) authority (Bergman, 1981).

Only after these preconditions are satisfied per nurse per patient can a nurse use authority to purposefully actualize outcomes. Therefore to make the relationship of care delivery methods to quality outcomes highly predictable and replicable, it is not the method but the accountability factor that must be established, developed, and constantly reinforced. According to Bergman (1981), "Nurses must move beyond 'talking about' accountability, and more into building specific measures, tools, periods and systems of reporting and implementing accountability" (p. 55).

QUESTIONS ABOUT EVALUATION

Because there has not been adequate investigation intrainstitutionally or otherwise to elucidate and define the outcomes that are a result of the nursing function, unfortunately it is premature to declare which care

Primary Nursing Structure

1. The Nurse Manager (NM) is accountable for assuring that every patient has a primary nurse upon or before admission/transfer or entry into the ambulatory area.

2. Each RN must carry a minimum of one primary patient at any given time.

3. Assignment of primary nurses will be based upon the nurse's time schedule, current caseload, and ability to independently carry out the nursing process required by the patient. Assignment of a primary nurse for orientation/professional development purposes will occur only when appropriate supervision can be provided.

4. The name of the primary nurse assigned to each patient will appear on the nursing assessment form, the patient's Kardex, the patient's chart, the patient's bedside card, or patient's clipboard on the door. In addition, a complete posting of the assignments of primary nurses and their patients will be in a central location on the unit. Each primary patient and family will be given a business card by their primary nurse.

5. Nurses who work permanent nights or less than four shifts per week will not ordinarily be assigned primary patients except under circumstances approved by the NM, i.e., there may be a situation where a part-time nurse may be a primary nurse for a patient who has a predictable short length of stay.

6. Daily patient assignments will be based upon each patient's individual requirements for varying levels of nursing care. Primary nurses will be responsible for the direct care of their patients whenever possible, especially if it facilitates successful completion of a nursing plan of care.

7. Primary nurses will communicate with associates, physicians, and other professionals involved in patient care through vehicles such as change of shift report, critical paths, physicians' rounds, multi-disciplinary care conferences, discharge planning rounds, and documentation.

8. Each unit will conduct patient care conferences as needed, designed for problem solving and educational purposes.

9. Primary nursing consultation sessions will be held weekly by the NM with the staff in each unit. They will be documented and submitted monthly to the nursing office. Primary nurses should request consultation as needed.

10. Off-duty involvement should be discouraged. The major responsibility of a nurse in this institution is to provide the highest quality of care to patients during scheduled hours on duty and to utilize the peer group on the nursing staff to continue care and support when the primary nurse is off duty. Other resources, e.g., volunteers, family, civic organizations, should appropriately be used in providing extra-hospital experience when these are desirable.

From New England Center Hospitals Department of Nursing. Used with permission.

delivery method is most predictive of quality. The methods cannot be compared side by side because neither the operational definition for primary nursing nor the expected results (beyond patient satisfaction levels) have been agreed upon. Role and process rather than product and effectiveness have been reviewed, with rather insufficient nongeneralizable results (Giovenetti, 1986).

The basic tenets of increased *autonomy, authority,* and *accountability* in the primary nurse's role appear to be universal among those who defined primary nursing (Manthey, 1973; Marram, 1974). The ubiquity of these concepts, however, *created the potential for a wide variety of applications.* Although some investigators provided lengthy descriptions of the primary nursing units, as well as those to which they were compared, others failed to provide any *operational definition* of primary nursing or any of the other organizational modes studied. *This omission represents the single most pervasive problem characterizing the research to date and makes virtually impossible any effort to provide a truly integrative analysis of the research.* Many investigators recognized this as a major limitation of their studies, and few investigators suggested that their results were generalizable.

Perhaps the only research that stretched past the usual philosophic approach to evaluating primary nursing was that of Jones (1975). She broke new ground by comparing clinical and financial outcomes (for patients receiving renal grafts) on a primary nursing unit with a nonprimary nursing unit in the same hospital. On a unit with primary nursing, patients receiving renal grafts had fewer "negative behaviors," 1.4 complications (compared with 4.6), a 28-day length of stay (compared with 46), and a cost of $61,000 less than for those on a nonprimary nursing floor.

Unfortunately, primary nursing, with its opportunities for professional growth of staff nurses and physical, emotional, and financial benefits for patients, remains an underutilized model. In the late 1960s, primary nursing was perceived as an emotional and a political choice rather than a standard for all nurses and patients. For nearly 25 years, its potential lay dormant in a majority of nursing departments. Although accountability and the fundamental role of the staff nurse were not developed, care delivery methods were affected by many influences: renovated units, new technologies, downsizing, and changes in supply and demand, to name a few. The current restructuring of health care services and reimbursement systems creates a much-needed catalyst for the advancement of professional nursing. Both care delivery methods and the role of the staff nurse in relation to quality are ready for analysis. In lieu of concrete, logical data, a definitive explicit work design must outline a pattern that supports an exact relationship between quality and delivery methods. Indeed, the equation between quality and delivery methods is not linear and dyadic but *triadic.* In it, nursing is not a service of tasks but rather a business with a product. According to Zander (1987, p. 1):

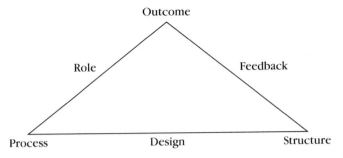

FIG 7-1 Relationship between quality and delivery method.

As in all businesses, nursing links the classic anchors of structure, process, and outcome in a dynamic organization of design, role, and feedback. *Design* is the way structural components (manpower, equipment, time) are expected to support the actual production processes. *Role* is the set of behaviors that is expected to transform the production process into an actual product. *Feedback* is the essential link between the outcomes of a system and the revisions and adaptations it must make to better do its work. The *care delivery method,* then, is the combination work design, role, and feedback components.

The relationships are illustrated in Fig. 7-1.

Without primary nursing, the role of a staff nurse is undifferentiated from other staff members and feedback is random. In terms of a musical analogy, nurses know the notes to play during their shifts (design) but not the entire piece of music. They are replaced by other musicians who play only their assigned notes, whereas the conductor (charge nurse, head nurse, or physician), hopefully, puts the concert together for the patient and family. It becomes clear that with this weakly constructed equation, nursing is not in control of its product—patient outcomes. Without control there can be no meaningful feedback or evaluation.

The next section outlines the evolution of a triadic equation describing primary nursing, managed care, and case management.

TOWARD PREDICTABILITY: PRIMARY NURSING AS THE CORE

Primary nursing was the first formal professional model in hospital nursing. The classic triad demonstrates that in a primary nursing model, *design* is the nursing care plan, *role* is the primary nurse (and associate), and *feedback* is audits of structure and process (charts, satisfaction, assignments, and so forth), as illustrated in Fig. 7-2.

The model for primary nursing is largely unit-based, implemented to achieve higher degrees of continuity and satisfaction for patients, their families, and their nurses. In addition, accountability for the outcomes of nursing care achievable while the patient is on a primary nurse's unit is a

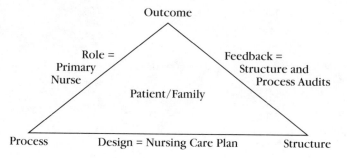

FIG 7-2 The classic triad of primary nursing.

key principle of the model. The attention on the accountability factor rather than on task responsibility has assisted many hospitals in developing a primary nursing care model that does not compromise professional standards yet stays flexible to the particular realities of the setting.

The primary nursing tradition includes all steps of the formal nursing process, caregiver as care planner, therapeutic primary nurse–patient/family relationships, patient education, communication, coordination, and collaboration among nursing staff members and disciplines. Indeed, the primary nurse must possess a blend of clinical, process, and management skills.

Primary nursing was the best model for professional practice until the industry turned its attention to case types in the form of DRGs. Because nursing is tied to all aspects of the patient's existence in hospitals, the changes in health care affect both nurses and their patients.

Increased percentages of acutely ill patients, decreased lengths of stay, and case-based management information and accounting systems create stress in even the most progressive, primary nursing departments. The pressure on nursing to justify its existence as a relatively expensive clinical component is ever present. To add to the confusion, the competition for more and more of a staff nurse's role, even by other nurses through the route of external case management, is increasing.

Historically, nurses have always managed care. In hospitals, however, their perspective usually is the management of care for the crisis, the shift, or the stay in a given geographic unit. Nurses still are seen, and perceive themselves, as task workers. Thus their authority is limited and their image is weak. Yet focused studies of nurses in practice reveal that nurses are highly outcome-oriented and effective in their interventions. In fact, one task may lead to three desirable clinical outcomes. The inherent strength of nursing, however, seems to be lost in roles that have enormous responsibilities but impoverished authority within the health care institution. Clearly, a stronger model that reformulates the role of the traditional primary nurse is needed. The model should keep professional nursing at the pivotal juncture of cost and quality and should empower the staff nurse to be truly accountable for the clinical and financial outcomes of nursing care throughout an entire episode of illness (Zander, 1987).

TRANSITION: MANAGED CARE

Managed care goes a step further in strengthening the equation between care delivery systems and quality. Managed care is a clinical system or process that, when used with any care delivery system, optimizes the achievement of standard clinical outcomes within fiscally responsible time frames. In other words, managed care actually is project management at the provider-client level. Managed care makes outcomes more predictable because the interventions of physicians, nurses, and providers from other key departments are negotiated, timed, and sequenced within overall standards of care for a specific case type.

Managed care in acute care settings is a six-staged clinical system that includes (1) the use of critical paths, (2) change-of-shift report given from the critical path format, (3) variance analysis every shift for every patient by every caregiver, (4) case consultation for variances, and (5) the regular use of health care team meetings. As a sixth step, data about variances are collected, aggregated, and evaluated by the head nurse as part of a quality improvement cycle.

The transition to managed care and the strengthening of the delivery method to improve the quality equation are outlined in the following paragraphs. Fig. 7-3 presents a graphic depiction of the transition.

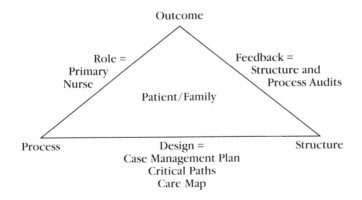

Care Map™ is a registered trademark of the Center for Nursing Case Management

FIG 7-3 Transition to managed care.

Care Plans to Case Management Plans, Critical Paths, and Care Maps*

The nursing care plans used during the past 25 years are weak tools for three main reasons. First, they lack guidelines that include collaboration with either patients or physicians. Second, they usually are not developed with any specific time lines or deadlines, and third, they are too conceptually oriented to provide many caregivers with clear directions. In addition, with the current fast pace of clinical care, the daily revision of care plans would be extremely difficult.

Since 1985, New England Medical Center Hospitals has been developing outcome-based collaborative tools for quality care within cost constraints. The master documents are entitled *Case Management Plans* (Table 7-1, pp. 98-99), and the abbreviated version is called a *Critical Path* (Fig. 7-4). Both are descriptive and prescriptive tools. When used as part of the complete managed care clinical system, they go a long way toward guaranteeing quality processes and outcomes. Besides being excellent management tools, they also assist with rapid orientation of new staff members. Their newest format, which combines both documents, is called a Care Map and can replace nursing care plans.

Primary Nurse Strengthened

Managed care strengthens the role of the primary nurse through a better work design, with responsibilities more equally distributed around the clock to all caregivers. Therefore, even though the primary nurse is accountable for the results of the care, there is a tighter directive for how these results will occur within an appropriate length of stay. Each RN and LPN focuses on the processes and outcomes every 8 hours. Nursing care and its quality are put into a context of outcomes and time.

To accomplish managed care, every nurse is educated about DRGs, how to formulate a critical path, how to give a report from a critical path, and how to recognize, evaluate, and act on patient variances in care. Thus, whether or not the primary nurse is present, all staff members have guidelines on which to anticipate physician action, organize and sequence events critical to a smooth hospital course, and inform patients and their families. In addition, the primary nurse receives case consultation from peers on a timely basis—before problems become serious, and is expected to organize and run health care team meetings. The critical path and unit-based systems such as the change-of-shift report supply more consistent continuity of the plan of care than does the traditional care plan.

Managed care is extremely valuable for units that have many part-time and float staff. Although the role of these staff members is not "primary," their role in relation to quality outcomes and processes *is* primary. Bower elaborates on this point (1988, p. 3):

*Care Map is a registered trademark of the Center for Nursing Case Management.

Patient _____

MD _____

Case Manager _____

Date Critical Path _____

Reviewed by MD _____

Date

Case Type Myocardial _____

Infarction _____

DRG ___ 122 ___

Expected LOS ___ 7 Days ___

**MYOCARDIAL INFARCTION
CRITICAL PATHWAY**

	Day 1	Day 2	Day 3	Day 4	Day 5	Day 6	Day 7
ICU			6S				
Consults		Cardiac Rehab. Dietician				Copy of Low Chol. No Added Salt Diet	
Tests	EKG	EKG · ETT if nec. for Day 6 Echo, Muga, if nec.	EKG Receive MBs R/I or R/O MI Holter if nec. on Day 5		Holter ETT Cath. if nec.		
Activity	BRP w/ Commode		OOB Chair		Amb in Rm/Hall w/Asst	Up Ad ———> Lib Stairs	
Treatments	O₂ ——————————————————> D/C O₂ Cardiac ——————————————————————————> Monitor I & O qd ——————————————————————————>					D/C Monitor p negative Holter D/C I & O qd wt, unless CHF	
Meds	IV ——————— Heparin ——————————————————————————> D/C Heparin Lock						Lock
Diet	No Added Salt, Low Chol. Diet ——>						
Discharge Planning			VNA		Check w/ Attending RE:D/C Date	Discharge Orders	Discharge before 12 Noon
Teaching	Angina, MI, PN., Med, Teaching Plan in Chart	Begin MI Teaching Plan	3 discharge classes Formal Med tx				Amb Classes Re:Risk Factors Diet & smoking

Admission Date _____   Discharge Date _____   Discharge Time _____

Days in ICU _____   Stress test date _____   Cardiac cath. date _____

Days in Routine bed _____   Thalium _____

Routine _____

Holter date _____

Copyright: New England Medical Center Hospitals 1987, Department of Nursing

DATE	VARIATION	CAUSE	ACTION TAKEN

(Reverse side of Critical Pathway form shown above)

FIG 7-4 Myocardial infarction critical pathway. (From New England Medical Center Hospitals, Department of Nursing. Copyright 1987. Used with permission.)

The contributions of part-time nurses, including floats, per diems, and agency nurses, become more outcome oriented. With increasing utilization of temporary and part-time nurses, it is important to find ways to incorporate their care into the overall picture of the patient's episode of illness. This is true for the patient as well as for the staff. With managed care, nurses who work on an intermittent basis can quickly determine what has happened to the patient in the past and what is needed during their shift to move the patient towards outcomes. As a result, there is less tendency to lose time with the patient as the nurse "catches up." In addition, the nurses feel more satisfied because they can readily see how their contributions during the shift fit into the patient's total care.

TABLE 7-1   Case Management Plan

Diagnosis: Stroke   **Length of stay:** 7 weeks
DRG: 14   **MDC***: 1   **Unit**: Rehabilitation

Problem	Outcome (The patient...)	Week	Intermediate Goal (The patient...)
Potential for complications/ self-care: 1. Inappropriate medication administration and/or side effects Risk factors: • Lack of knowledge • Lack of skill	For participants in self-medication program: • And/or significant other accurately and independently administers own medications All other patients: • States rationale for prescribed treatment • Accurately states the prescribed medication regimen: (i.e., action dose, frequency and side effects for each discharge medication)	4 6 0-7 4-7	• Accurately states the prescribed medication regimen and its rationale • States medica- tion, action dose, fre- quency and side effects for each discharge medication • Completes medication teaching plan • And/or signifi- cant other participates in medication teaching
2. Injury Risk factors: • Sensory deficits • Altered mobility • Lack of knowledge • Environmental condition	• Does not experience preventable bodily harm	1-7 5-7 7	• Actively par- ticipates in rehab program gram in antic- ipation of pass and eventual discharge • Completes pass evalua- tion form • States com- munity ser- vices which will be avail- able

From New England Medical Center Hospitals' Department of Nursing; © 1987.
*MDC, Main diagnostic category.

Week	Process (The nurse...)	Week	Process (The physician...)
2-3	• Initiates medication teaching plan • Reviews this with family • Provides medication cards to patients/ family	4 4	• Stabilizes medication regimen. Weans any unnecessary meds • Orders self-meds if patient is a candidate for self-med program
4-7	• Reinforces content of medication teaching plan with patient/ family		
1	• Assesses patient as a candidate for self-meds • Follows policy on self-meds		
4	• Initiates teaching of discharge meds to patient/significant other		
4	• Provides medication cards to patient/ significant other		
4-7	• Reinforces medication teaching		
7	• Arranges appropriate follow-up with community resources for Coumadin		
2	• Collaborates with team to identify discharge date		
2	• Collaborates with patient to identify disposition and potential environmental barriers		
4	• Prepares patient for day pass		
5	• Prepares patient/ family for weekend pass		

Structure and Process Surveys to Outcome Audits

It is the feedback loop between outcomes and structure that is the least developed in all care delivery systems. In primary nursing alone, the feedback loop often comprises either postdischarge letters from patients and families or satisfaction surveys of nurses and patients. Although useful, these methods are not as formal as are needed by health care institutions that have to make difficult choices about money, quality, and personnel. In addition, feedback for the action being reviewed must be as immediate as possible to affect patient outcomes. As a result, postdischarge feedback is not timely for improving quality during the care episode.

Therefore comprehensive and concurrent audits that measure the structures, processes, *and* outcomes believed to be imperative to the care delivery method must be developed (McKenna, 1991). In managed care the processes and outcomes are monitored each shift. In addition to the nursing caregiver who is monitoring expected quality, selected patients also are using copies of their critical path to participate in their care. The whole managed care process ensures the rapid identification and correction of variances that have potential quality implications.

Variance analysis increases the fund of clinical knowledge not only about one patient but about groups of patients. As the nurse manager (or group practice in case management) tracks these collective variances, new patterns of interventions and programs can be instituted. In the past, these new ideas might have taken longer to crystalize because the quality review usually took place in retrospect. With managed care, quality review is immediate, and the current patient receives maximum benefit.

In summary, managed care puts the clinician through a series of questions for each patient that always should be asked but often is lost in the fast pace and fragmentation of today's clinical settings. These questions are fundamental to the management of cost and quality outcomes:

What should happen?
What is actually happening?
What didn't happen and why?
What can be done about it?
Who can rectify it and how?

According to Zander (1988b), "Managed care provides care givers with better management tools and systems than previously available. It is a mindset and a technology that is neither computer nor person/personality dependent" (p. 3).

NURSING CASE MANAGEMENT

Nursing case management further clarifies and enhances the equation of care delivery methods and quality by providing patients and families with a group of nurse (RN)–physician caregivers who manage quality throughout an entire episode of illness. Although managed care revises unit-based tools and activities, case management changes roles and relationships. As managed care strengthens the design, case management strengthens the roles of the principal caregivers, and research will strengthen feedback.

Nursing case management can best be described as a matrix model at the caregiver level, creating a "unit without walls." In it, specific staff primary nurses are in formally trained groups with other primary nurses throughout the hospital who take within their case assignments specific case types of specific physicians. If every patient in an institution is receiving managed care, then case management is a logical "next step" for providing tighter quality controls for patients whose conditions place them at medical or financial high risk.

It can be seen in the "ground rules" (see box on p. 102) that nursing case management is not a care delivery system but is related to the care delivery system in that it structures certain nurses as caregivers when certain kinds of patients of certain physicians are on their units. For example, if Mr. Z had a stroke, he would have one of three physicians, and his primary nurses would be Paul D in the emergency room, Barbara W in the neurology ICU (if needed), Monica U on the neurology floor, Mary B in rehabilitation, and outpatient follow-up by Tricia C. These nurses would give Mr. Z care whenever on duty and would trust their peers to continue quality care through the use of critical paths by means of managed care. The group of nurses meet weekly to review their roster of acutely ill patients and meet with the attending physician monthly to discuss stroke-related policies. With case-managed patients, the group practices reviews variances and recommends overall changes.

The advances in the equation of care delivery methods and quality are illustrated in Fig. 7-5 and the following paragraphs. Although imperfect, case management promises powerful improvements.

Case management plans and critical paths to contracts. "Better-briefed" patients is one of the 10 most powerful tactics for improving service quality in hospitals, according to the 1988 report of the Health Care Advisory Board (1988). Patient information about the expected course of hospitalization is as vital as education about the illness itself. As patients and families perceive group practices working on important outcomes, informing them and involving them at key junctures, the perception of quality increases.

Critical paths and case-management plans lend confidence to clinicians as to the content and timing of their communications with patients and families. Eventually, this security could lead to verbal if not written contracts.

Primary nurse-to-group practices. Each primary nurse in a group practice is part of the regular staffing of his or her unit. Primary nurses take

---

Ground Rules for Case Management

1. Every designated patient will be admitted to a formally-prepared group practice composed of an attending physician and staff nurses from each of the units and clinics likely to receive those patients.
2. All nurses in the group practice will give direct care as the patient's primary or associate nurse while the patient is on his/her geographic unit.
3. Every group practice will assign one of its nursing members to be the case manager who works with the attending physician in evaluating an individualized Case Management Plan (CMP) and Critical Path for each patient.
4. A Critical Path for the whole episode of care will be used to manage the care of every designated patient, both at change-of-shift report and during group practice meetings.
5. The nurses in the group practice will meet on a weekly basis at a consistent time and place and maintain a patient roster.
6. Each nurse member of the group practice will communicate immediate patient care issues with the attending physician while the patient is on his/her own unit. The assigned case manager will work through the group and the attending physician for non-emergent issues.
7. Negative variances from Critical Paths and/or CMPs require discussion with the attending physician, and a case management consultation when necessary.
8. The group practice will meet to discuss care patterns, policies, specific patients and variances, research questions and updated knowledge at their own predetermined intervals, e.g., monthly, bi-monthly. Minutes will be taken for reference by members who cannot attend.
9. Nurse members of the group practice will negotiate a flexible schedule that accommodates the needs of their case-managed patients and collaborative practices, *as well as* the needs of their units.
10. Responsibility of the case manager begins at notification of patient's entry into the system and ends with a formal transfer of accountability to the patient, family, another health care provider, or another institution.

From New England Medical Center Hospitals, © 1988. Used with permission.

certain kinds of patients within their shift responsibilities and primary case load. Exactly how these care delivery decisions are made depends on volume, training requirements, and other factors that influence any unit. The authority base of the staff primary nurse, however, is greatly increased by the knowledge and team building that are part of a required 3-day curriculum. Authority is further enhanced by the institutional sanction of case management and each group practice's explicit mission.

Audits to research. As case management plans and critical paths become validated and revised, we learn much about the causal relationship of process to outcomes. There is an enormous amount of research needed in many areas, including potential problems, the prevention of complications, the acquisition of self-care skills, and the experience of

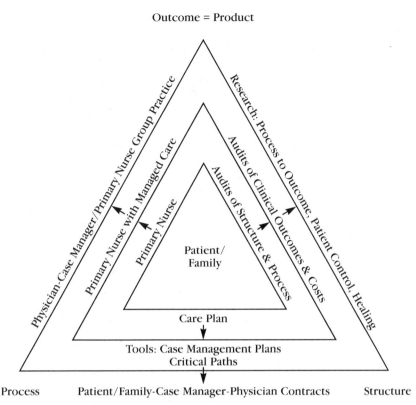

FIG 7-5 The professional advances of nursing case management (outcome = product).

being healed. At present, there appears to be more consensus among nurses about clinical outcomes than there is about diagnoses. Perhaps this is a clue to the unification of the collective strength in professional nursing.

To date, nursing care management has begun to accomplish at least five crucial goals (Stetler & DeZell, 1987):

1. To achieve "expected" or "standardized" outcomes
2. To promote collaborative practice, coordinated care, and continuity of care
3. To promote appropriate and reduced utilization of resources
4. To facilitate "early" discharge or discharge within an "appropriate" length of time
5. To promote professional development and satisfaction

CONCLUSION

What can be concluded about delivery systems and quality? First, the simpler the work design, the more empowered the caregiver. Second, the more immediate the feedback, the better the quality of processes and outcomes.

Health care institutions are complex systems with constantly changing variables. The care delivery method of the hour must be more a choreography than a march. It must have a pattern, but it must be resilient. Its theme is based on the premise that for each patient there must be a nurse directing, evaluating, and held accountable for the results of all the care given.

Without primary nursing or case management, or both, quality care still can be achieved, but predictability and accuracy of the chosen delivery method will be weak. Managed care can increase the design side of the equation, thus improving continuity across all shifts and more consistent attainment of outcome. Either managed care with primary nursing or case management as described here, however, remains the patient's best road to quality care in every sense of the word.

REFERENCES

Bergman, B. (1981). Accountability—Definition and dimensions. *International Nursing Review, 29*(2), 55.

Bower, K. (1988). Managed care: Controlling costs, guaranteeing outcomes. *Definition, 3*(3), 3.

Giovenetti, P. (1986). Evaluation of primary nursing. *Annual Review of Nursing Research, 4,* 128-129.

Health Care Advisory Board. (1988). *Service quality at U.S. hospitals: 24 tactics for improving hospital service* (Vol. 1). Washington, DC: The Advisory Board Co.

Jones, K. (1975). Study documents effects of primary nursing on renal transplant patients. *Hospitals, 49*(24), 85-89.

Manthey, M. (1973). Primary nursing is alive and well in the hospital. *American Journal of Nursing, 73,* 83-87.

Marram, G. D. (1974). *Primary nursing.* St. Louis: C. V. Mosby.

McKenna, M. (1991). Patient discharge outcome audits: Improving quality and reducing cost. *Definition, 6*(1), 1-3.

Stetler, C., & DeZell, A. D. (1987). *Nursing case management: Designs for transformation.* Boston: New England Medical Center Hospitals.

Zander, K. (1987). Nursing case management: A classic. *Definition, 2*(2), 1.

Zander, K. (1988a). Nursing case management: Resolving the DRG paradox. *Nursing Clinics of North America, 23*B, 504.

Zander, K. (1988b). Why managed care works. *Definition, 3*(4), 3.

CHAPTER 8

Total Quality Management in Health Care

Ellen Marszalek-Gaucher

Total quality management is a proactive approach to quality assurance that focuses on the continuous improvement of quality and the reduction of wasteful resource expenditures. A customer focus, a problem-solving approach, and teamwork are necessary factors in implementation. The approach has been used successfully by nurses and has a number of positive implications for health care workers and for the organization. This chapter describes the concept and its implementation in one hospital setting.

It is likely that the nineties will become known as the decade of renewed commitment to quality in health care. Executives of health care organizations are recognizing that a major quality transformation is required to compete successfully. The drive to transform comes from pressures internal and external to the health care industry. After two decades of growth, limited financial risk, and administrative autonomy, we have entered a period with new ground rules and incentives that challenge the financial viability of most health care organizations. These new incentives have increased competition in an industry already overburdened with the restructuring required to adapt to changing medical practice and the explosion of new technology. The challenge to

University of Michigan Medical Center, 300 North Ingalls, Ann Arbor, MI 48109.

Series on Nursing Administration — Volume III, 1992

today's health care executive is to deliver high-quality care at a reasonable price.

Enhancing health care quality is a difficult task; as Berwick (1988) points out, "Healthcare because of its complexity and special sociology has lagged behind other industries in the development of tools to measure and control quality" (p. 14). Although we pride ourselves on being experts in traditional quality assurance, we have often been satisfied with treating the symptoms of poor quality rather than the disease. We have defined quality in a narrow sense, focusing on the structure, process, and more recently the outcomes of care. Measures such as mortality rates, infection rates, and other complications of care focus on negative results. Other measures such as repeat hospitalization or surgical procedures focus on recidivism. In both cases these are negative measures of quality. On the other hand, the total quality approach focuses on meeting the valid requirements of the customer, a more positive measure.

Our method of improving health care quality in the past has been by inspection. The goal of inspection is to remove unacceptable services, products, or information on the back end by finding the defective services and revising them. Inspection always costs an organization more money. The total-quality philosophy encourages quality through prevention and design. Prevention is the approach of improving systems on the front end by designing quality into the service. This reduces the cost of poor quality. In addition to reducing costs quality planning enhances revenues.

A NEW DEFINITION OF QUALITY

It seems obvious that to solve the quality-cost problems in health care requires a move from a reactive to a proactive system. Successful industries have shown us that implementation of total quality will mean better customer satisfaction, smoother working relationships within the organization, decreased cost, improved productivity and staff morale, and an ability to compete more effectively. The word "total" is used to indicate the drive to continuously improve all products and services everywhere in the organization. Total quality may well be the dawn of a new era for health care, one where we move from attempting to ensure quality to actually measuring and improving the quality of all products and services.

The implementation of total quality requires first a vision, a new sense of purpose and direction that is shared among all employees in the organization. Second, it demands a commitment throughout the organization to learn new skills and an amalgamation of tools and techniques that support continuous improvement. Everyone in the organization must learn to manage with facts. Third, total quality requires the utilization of teams and the team spirit for problem solving, as each employee participates in improving his or her job and the organization as a whole. Finally and most important, total quality requires that the organization be customer driven; in other words the organization focuses its efforts on identifying and satisfying the requirements of the customers.

The New Quality Philosophy

Where did this new philosophy spring from? Many credit the current resurgence of interest in quality to June of 1980 when W. Edwards Deming appeared in an NBC documentary called *If Japan Can, Why Can't We?* It compared the productivity in Japan with productivity in the United States and showed the progress toward meeting quality goals achieved by the Japanese over several decades. The message was clear; this new quality commitment and intense listening to customers had allowed Japan to become a dominant player in the emerging global marketplace. Corporate America heard the message, and many chief executive officers in the United States began to use these same quality tools and concepts to enable their organizations to more closely meet customer requirements. Corporations such as Ford Motor Company, IBM, Xerox, Motorola, and Florida Power and Light have used these techniques to enhance quality and to improve both quality of work life and bottom-line results.

In the late 1980s, health care organizations began to implement total quality initiatives. The University of Michigan Medical Center participated in a National Demonstration Project (NDP) sponsored by the John A. Hartford Foundation and the Harvard Community Health Plan. The purpose of this project was to advance the state of the art in health care quality control. Each of the 21 participating health care organizations was paired with a quality expert from industry to learn how to apply the tools and techniques of total quality management to a specific project. The NDP enjoyed great success, many of the organizations made substantial progress with the project, and a large proportion made the decision to implement total quality management. A recent study (Kratochwill, 1990) found that of the original 21 participating organizations, 17 identified formal total quality improvement plans. The plans of the organizations with programs in place varied considerably, ranging from searching for a consultant to fully implementing in-house instruction. Nearly all the organizations stated that the current environment of fiscal and quality pressures on health care organizations will ensure that total quality will be further tested and modified throughout the health care industry. Although long-term results are not yet available, Laffel (1990) indicates that "about 100 health care organizations are experimenting with total quality management science. Early results suggest that quality management is applicable to most, if not all, aspects of patient care and related services" (p. 30).

Quality Gurus

Several gurus of quality have emerged. Deming and Joseph Juran both traveled to Japan after World War II to teach the concepts of statistical quality control and continuous improvement to the Japanese. Deming's approaches were so successful in helping to create a revolution for quality in Japan that the Union of Japanese Scientists and Engineers (JUSE) initiated the annual Deming Prize, Japan's most prestigious quality award, to honor him. Feigenbaum, the author of *Total Quality Control* (1983), proposed this concept as a system for integrating quality efforts to meet customers' needs. Although each of these specialists recommends a slightly different approach, the basic philosophies are the same. Scientific thinking needs to occur at all levels of the organization to facilitate continuous improvement.

THE TOTAL QUALITY PROCESS

Total quality is a means of ensuring customer satisfaction by involving every employee in improving the quality of every product and service in the organization. It means evaluating all systems and processes and improving them. With quality improvement everyone benefits: the organization, the worker, and society (Fig. 8-1). The total quality process provides a framework for organizations to design quality services, to monitor their progress, and to focus on continuous improvement.

The significant amount of rework and waste in health care adds cost to the system. This is termed the *cost of poor quality*. Total quality management is a way to reduce waste and rework the process so that quality failures do not happen. An example of this concept can be illustrated by a look at the patient education required for diagnostic testing. If there is quality planning, the patient arrives well prepared for the examination, and the test proceeds. If, on the other hand, the patient received faulty instructions and comes in poorly prepared, the test may have to be rescheduled. This is a quality failure, with costs related to the poor quality. It creates scheduling problems for the organization because of the need to reschedule and results in the loss of revenue and time. The patient may lose an extra day of work and suffer anxiety because of the rescheduling and the ultimate delay in diagnosis. Neither the customer nor the organization is pleased. The worst-case scenario is that the customer will lose confidence in the organization and not return. Quality planning, by ensuring that the test proceeds appropriately, allows resources to be allocated to areas of true need rather than to correcting failures.

Customer Focus

Total quality programs require a commitment to the customer, both those internal and those external to the organization. The following image is a helpful way to conceptualize the relationship of customers and suppliers: "for any transaction involving a product, service, or information, the person or the organization at the tail of the arrow is the

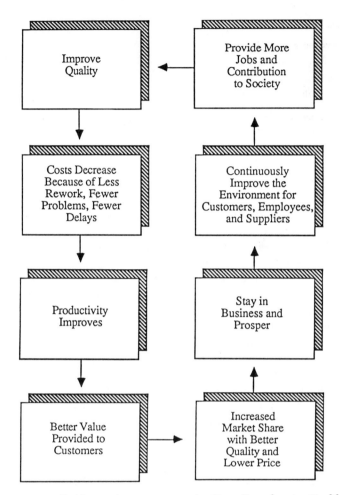

FIG 8-1 Continuous improvement cycle. (From *Transforming Health Care Organizations*, Figure 8, page 85. © 1990 Jossey-Bass, Inc. Publishers, San Francisco, CA. Used with permission.)

supplier, and the person or organization at head of the arrow is the customer'' (Marszalek-Gaucher & Coffey, 1990, p. 85) (Fig. 8-2).

Internal customers are the people in the next department, such as the unit clerk or the patient transporter. How many times do we ask ourselves: What does the person next in line need from me to be successful? If I am a supplier, have I told the unit clerk to communicate to the transporter all the information needed to facilitate a smooth trip to physical therapy? Perhaps the patient has had a poor night and has not had much sleep because of pain. Perhaps the transporter needs to know to bring a stretcher instead of a wheelchair or that the visit needs to be timed after pain medication. Unless the customer is provided with the

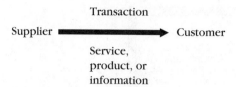

FIG 8-2 Total quality transactions. (From *Transforming Health Care Organizations,* Figure 8, page 85. © 1990 Jossey-Bass, Inc. Publishers, San Francisco, CA. Used with permission.)

correct information, the procedure may fall into the category of a quality failure. Understanding requirements allows accurate communication to take place and results in a more efficient, cost-effective process.

Understanding the customer/supplier relationship. There are many external customers in health care: patients, families, referring physicians, other health care professionals, third-party payers, and regulatory agencies. The list seems endless. In the past most external customers were excluded from formal processes to define quality because health care providers believed recipients did not have appropriate information to make decisions. Today's health care consumers are much more sophisticated and are demanding that their requirements be taken into consideration. For example, General Motors Corporation, as a purchaser of health care services, recently terminated contracts with six HMOs that did not meet its requirements for quality and cost. Clearly those health care organizations that do not respond to the requirements of customers may find their ability to compete significantly altered.

Determining customer needs and expectations is a complicated task. Each department within the institution must first identify its customers, perhaps by a brainstorming exercise at a staff meeting, and then talk directly to those customers to determine their requirements. Quality plans must then be established to align the department to meet these needs. Frequent checking with the customers allows the organization to measure progress.

Listening to the voice of the customer. For health care organizations, shifting to a true customer focus requires the development of a new way of thinking. We must learn to listen more effectively to our customers. This sounds like an easy task, but it can be extremely traumatic. To improve services the nursing service at the University of Michigan Hospitals (UMH) held a focus session with patients and families who had complained about their nursing care. According to the director of nursing, "it was very painful to listen to the patient's stories of failure; it hurts when you realize needs aren't being met." After the testimonials, the audience of nurses and customers broke up into small groups to plan for quality improvement. The results were amazingly positive, and the customers and the nurses left the session reassured that the quality failures would not be repeated. This is the essence of total quality: listening to the customer and making adjustments.

Quality Indicators

Once customers' requirements are known, quality indicators that measure the ability to meet these requirements need to be developed. These indicators need to be monitored on a monthly basis. At UMH, to measure our customers' response we have chosen institutional quality indicators in five areas. Key customer groups are patients, referring physicians, payers, employees and medical staff, and students.

Each department also must develop quality indicators specific to that department and measure those on a monthly basis. Continuous measurement allows needed service adjustments to be identified before quality failures occur.

Teamwork

Teams are the building blocks of total quality. The work of improvement is done by those closest to the process who have the knowledge necessary to make the changes needed. In health care we think we know all about teams. This belief stems from the fact that health care professionals work as a team to save lives. I have observed, however, that after the patient care crisis is over, the professionals who have worked so well together retreat back to their professional turf. Under normal circumstances the communication patterns change and barriers surface until action is required for the next crisis.

Through total quality tools and techniques people learn to establish a common language that allows team members to share their knowledge. Utilizing the seven quality tools teaches members how to display data graphically and how to identify problems and potential solutions rather than just talk about problems. Total quality is an information-driven process, a process that keeps people from jumping to conclusions as they learn to focus on finding the root cause of problems. Teaching employees to identify and use facts means moving from a crisis-oriented organization to a planning-oriented organization. The use of the Shewhart cycle (Deming, 1986), or the plan, do, check, act (P-D-C-A) cycle illustrated in Fig. 8-3, means studying the planned change, trying the change on an experimental or test basis, checking to see if results followed the predicted hypothesis, and, if successful, acting to standardize the result in daily practice. The expected results then become the standards against which future performance is measured to ensure that results gained are retained.

Managers traditionally have been trained to perform the plan, check, and act activities, leaving only the do, or actual work function, to the employee. This is consistent with the scientific management theory of Fredrick Taylor in 1920s. This style of management removed the ability

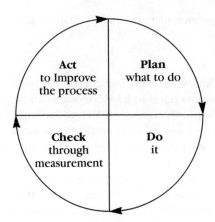

FIG 8-3 P-D-C-A cycle.

to improve processes from the person with the greatest impact on the outcome — the employee doing the work. Through teams and application of the P-D-C-A cycle, control over the process is turned to the employee. As a result, total quality empowers employees to continuously improve processes.

Impact on nursing. Quality improvement teams in nursing have worked on such opportunities as quality of care issues, staffing issues, and quality of work life issues. They have worked on issues within nursing (functional teams) or on cross-functional teams, dealing with issues such as patient transportation. We have found that nurses are adept at learning and applying total quality tools and techniques. The National Demonstration Project also reported success within other nursing groups. Berwick, Blanton, & Roessner (1990, p. 149) made the following observations and comments:

> Among the happiest of findings was the receptivity of nurses in hospitals to the methods of quality improvement. Many of the project team leaders reported that nurses became champions for these methods faster than most other staff groups. We do not yet know why, but it may involve the "process-mindedness" that is at the core of quality management. To comprehend processes, one must be able to see the interdependencies that all processes contain. The professional training of nurses may help them to see what they and others do in process terms, thus clearing the way for efforts to gather specific information on processes.

Another reason nurses have been successful with the total quality process is that P-D-C-A closely resembles the nursing process, a tool nurses have used for years to plan and deliver nursing care, as illustrated in Fig. 8-4. The scientific problem-solving method already is part of nursing care.

One of our successful nursing teams has been the UMH surgical ICU

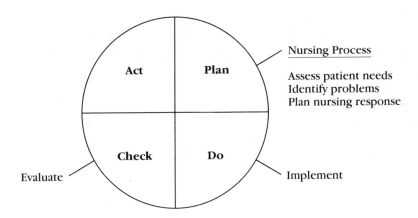

FIG 8-4 P-D-C-A and the nursing process.

team, which developed an opportunity list that consisted of issues of importance to them. These issues included differentiating practice, unit organization, pod clustering, workload monitoring, and employee work scheduling. The first project the team chose to work on was differentiating practice. Team members included the nurse manager, the medical director of the unit, and staff nurses. They identified three major questions for consideration: What provider mix would promote quality patient care? Can the surgical intensive care unit (SICU) recruit and develop the number of qualified staff needed to continue practicing in an all-RN framework? Can society afford an all-RN system? The analysis included brainstorming issues related to differentiating practice, research of the literature, and consultation with experts in the field. Developing consensus about the definition of professional practice and a list of delegable activities generated considerable debate. From these meetings the team determined the need for alternate care providers and developed a job description for a new category of ICU worker. They interviewed candidates and selected the pool of candidates for the pilot project. The pilot was highly successful, and alternate providers are being permanently added to the staff in incremental steps. The team has moved to the next priority item and is now studying unit organization.

Quality improvement teams. Quality improvement teams at UMH may choose their own issue or may have an issue assigned to them. The teams follow a standard problem-solving method and document the steps taken on a "storyboard," which is posted in the department for everyone to see and comment on. The storyboard is a development of the Florida Power and Light Quality Process (Fig. 8-5). The process includes the following steps:

1. *Reason for improvement.* The team identifies a theme or problem area and the reason for working on it.

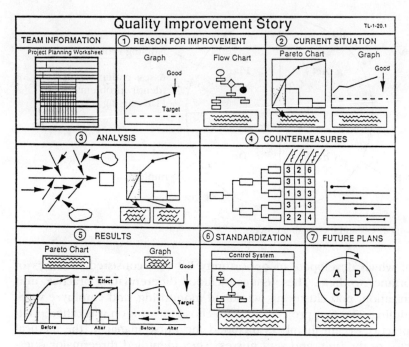

FIG 8-5 The storyboard. (From "QI Story," *TEAM LEADER COURSE.* © 1990 QUALTEC Quality Services Inc., Palm Beach Garden, FL. Used with permission.)

2. *Current situation.* The team selects a specific problem, writes a clear problem statement, and sets a target for improvement.
3. *Analysis.* Here the team identifies and verifies the root causes of the problem.
4. *Countermeasures.* At this step the proposed solutions or counter-measures are selected by the team to correct the root cause(s) of the problem.
5. *Results.* This step confirms that the problem and its root causes have been decreased and that the target for improvement has been met.
6. *Standardization.* This step allows the team to prevent the problem and its root causes from recurring.
7. *Future plans.* Here the team documents the next priority area for improvement.

The storyboard is a way to both document and share information relative to the team's effort.

Another example of a team effort that improved a process was increasing the nursing department's nursing resource pool (NRP) at UMH. Historically, head nurses of the inpatient units could request supplemental staffing either from external agencies or from the UMH supplemental staffing office NRP. Most head nurses contracted with the external agencies because the internal office traditionally did not meet their needs. When a new manager was appointed, she adopted a total quality approach and set up a team to study the problems of the NRP. The team interviewed all the customers to determine priorities and requirements. On the basis of investigation and input, many countermeasures were taken, including the development of new policies and procedures for staff assignments and categories. The size of the pool grew from 40 to 230 full-time equivalents. The customers assisted in the reformation of the NRP. Through meeting customer requirements the institution realized savings of approximately $4 million and reduced costs by 50% as the use of the internal NRP replaced outside agencies. Today requirements and needs are assessed on a monthly basis. The service has improved remarkably, the UMH program is the program of choice, and the customers are pleased (Marszalek-Gaucher & Coffey, 1990).

Employee Empowerment

Employee empowerment and involvement is a key principle in total quality. Only by encouraging the persons who are closest to the work to share their thoughts on how to improve the process can revolutionary change occur. Many times managers and supervisors are too far removed from the process to know how to make significant change. Effort must be spent in creating the kind of environment in which ideas are solicited and acted upon. Many times in health care there are more idea stoppers than idea supporters. By virtue of our professional training and desire to do no harm to patients we become "risk adverse." We all must learn new ways to bring forward ideas and to act on them. We must learn to develop more trusting and open environments in which teams can flourish.

Training

Training for total quality must include skill building in statistical thinking, customer orientation, effective teamwork, and ways to enhance creativity and innovation. There are several phases of the process, and each requires a different type of curriculum. The first phase is awareness; during this phase general exposure to the concepts is required. Learning about the history and philosophy of total quality is essential. Exposure to examples of successful projects from health care gives people a sense of the possible. In the second phase the learners need to understand the tools and techniques of total quality. Exposure to the concepts of variation, process capability, and the roles of the team members is necessary. The third phase is implementation. At this phase the team process is taught, along with documentation and reporting skills. The last phase is integration. In this phase the participants refine skills and weave total quality in the fabric of their work and therefore into the organization.

Managers at all levels, from the executives to first-line supervisors, need additional training to implement a total-quality approach. Total quality requires that managers learn how to be coaches and mentors. They must move from merely managing to leading the implementation of the new philosophy. Total quality requires risk taking and solicitation of ideas from all parts of the organization.

Training is a never-ending responsibility. New knowledge requires new programs to share learning throughout the organization. Ongoing training also helps employees to retain complex material. Finally, total quality must be integrated into new employee orientation to ensure that all new employees are ready to join quality improvement teams and to participate in generating ideas to improve quality. Consideration also should be given to including quality as a responsibility on all job descriptions, which would effectively establish a commitment to quality at the beginning of the employee's tenure with the organization.

Benchmarking

Total quality requires knowledge about the service quality provided by other organizations. Benchmarking allows one to survey the competition to look at customer satisfaction and reactions and to develop targets for improvement. Xerox was one of the first American companies to use this strategy. They developed four basic questions (Garvin 1988, p. 31):

1. Is the competition better? If so how much?
2. Why are they better?
3. What can we learn from them?
4. And how can we apply what we have learned to our business?

How many times have we asked these questions about nurses in a competing hospital. What changes would we make in practice if we began to ask these questions?

Benchmarking does not eliminate the need to keep improving, because customer expectations change and the competition may well learn by the competitor's success and begin to emulate that success. Hospitals have always compared themselves to the hospital across town or perhaps to the ones most like themselves in the state. The concept of benchmarking suggests we compare ourselves not just to other hospitals but to other successful businesses. Are our reception clerks equal to clerks in a fine hotel? How does our billing system compare with that of a quality business in our area or in the country? Does our food service compare with that of a restaurant? Does our nursing unit provide the same level of service competing hospitals provide? Benchmarking requires developing a quality plan to improve to that level. Goals for satisfaction with nursing services should be set at one or two levels higher than the competition. The goal is to delight the customer. The goal of continuous improvement means setting targets higher and higher to achieve new levels of quality.

REQUIREMENTS OF NURSES AND CUSTOMER

As nurses we believe we have been in touch with our customer's requirements. We are so close to the ultimate customer, the patient. Yet have we really understood customer requirements? A recent article in *Health Care Forum Journal* (Chapman, 1990), written by a former district attorney who now is a hospital administrator, concluded that many practices within health care are similar to prison practices. The author suggests that we take action now to treat patients as independent, autonomous partners in their own care and controllers of their own destiny and that each of us work actively for deinstitutionalization of the patient experience. Answers to the following questions may be revealing. Which practices in your organization or unit support the concept of an autonomous partnership? Do you view the family as part of the process or a barrier to providing the care you believe is necessary? What steps can your hospital take to enhance hospitalization? The first step may be to establish exit interviews with patients and families after discharge to ascertain their requirements and areas in which improvement is needed.

What about other consumers of nursing, pharmacy, materials management, or dietary services or clients of nurses in ambulatory or home care nursing? How well do we understand the interfaces, the places where we hand the patient to the next person in line? How effective have we been in viewing ourselves as customers or suppliers of service? The goal of total quality is to have a seamless organization in which no interdepartmental barriers or finger pointing occurs, in which systems work smoothly without flaws.

For many years we have read of the culture shock that occurs when new, energetic, idealistic students become nurses and enter nursing practice. Most times the shock occurs when new nurses realize that they have little control over professional practice and that autonomy in decision making rarely exists. They discover that much nursing practice consists of nonnursing, nonpatient care–oriented duties that take nurses away from the job they were hired to perform.

The total quality process allows ideas about practice improvement to come from the practitioner. One of the staff nurses from the UMH surgical ICU quality improvement team told an audience of about 50 administrators that for the first time in her career she felt a sense of control over her practice, that she and her team members were designing the model of the future for their unit, and that they were using the skills and education they had never before been able to use.

CONCLUSION

Although total quality sounds like common sense and good business practice, it is a complex process that will require many years and much effort to implement. Changing the culture of an organization to an environment characterized by trust and employee involvement is a monumental task. On the other hand, the rewards certainly are worth the effort. By addressing quality issues and streamlining systems and processes, we can reduce the cost of health care and allocate scarce resources more effectively. Utilizing total quality techniques within nursing may allow us to return control of practice to those doing the work and contribute to enhanced professionalism and job satisfaction.

UMH's total quality process began in 1987. Recognizing the power of the process, we are now trying to integrate it into every facet of our operations, both clinical and nonclinical. We are convinced that total quality is an investment in our people and our future. Each employee who contributes ideas, talents, and skills will ensure that UMH has the best chance for future success.

REFERENCES

Berwick, D. (1988). Measuring healthcare quality, *Pediatrics in Review, 10*(1), 14.

Berwick, D. M., Blanton, G. A., & Roessner, J. (1990). *Curing health care: New strategies for quality improvement.* San Francisco: Jossey-Bass.

Chapman, E. (1990, November/December). Hospitals and prisons. *Health Care Forum Journal.*

Deming, W. E. (1986). *Out of the crisis.* Cambridge: Center for Advanced Engineering Study, Massachusetts Institute of Technology.

Feigenbaum, A. V. (1983). *Total quality control.* New York: McGraw-Hill.

Garvin, D. (1988). *Managing quality.* New York: Collier-Macmillan.

Kratochwill, E. (1990). *National demonstration project on industrial quality control and health care quality: The progress in total quality of the original 21 participating organizations.* Unpublished manuscript, The University of Michigan Hospitals, Ann Arbor.

Laffel, G. (1990). Implementing quality management in health care: The challenges ahead. *Quality Progress,* November, p. 30.

Marszalek-Gaucher, E., & Coffey, R. J. (1990). *Transforming healthcare organizations.* San Francisco: Jossey-Bass.

CHAPTER 9

Community Nursing Care and Quality

Anne Rooney

The expansion of home health care has been accompanied by increased concern about the quality of care provided by home care agencies. Three agencies that examine and accredit these organizations are the National HomeCaring Council, the Community Health Accreditation Program of the National League for Nursing, and the Joint Commission on Accreditation of Healthcare Organizations. Each of these organizations has developed its own standards and procedures for accreditation. Efforts to ensure the quality of home care also have been undertaken by individual agencies. Evaluation of home care quality can be expected to remain a major concern during the next decade.

In the past century, community health nursing has experienced tremendous growth and challenge. From its origins, which focused primarily on maternal and child care and health promotion within the community, this component of nursing practice has expanded to encompass a spectrum of services. These services range from health promotion activities in a community clinic or county health department to case management services of elderly persons in the community to "high-tech" home health services such as home dialysis, ventilator management, and

Joint Commission on Accreditation of Healthcare Organizations, One Renaissance Boulevard, Oakbrook Terrace, IL 60181.

infusion therapy. In the past decade the impact of cost-containment strategies and prospective payment has increasingly shifted health care services from institutions to the community setting.

This trend in health policy occurs in a climate of increasing public demand for quality services in all health care settings, and community health nursing is not exempt. Consumers, regulatory bodies, the business community, payers, accrediting bodies, and the nursing profession itself have had a hand in shaping the present and future course of community health nursing. Indeed, even the American Bar Association's Commission on Legal Problems of the Elderly expressed serious concerns about the current state of quality in home health care to the House Select Committee on Aging in their 1986 report entitled *The Black Box of Home Care Quality*. This report surveyed existing Medicare and practice standards but concluded that such standards focused more on an organization's capability to deliver adequate care rather than on the quality of the care actually provided. The report by the American Bar Association (ABA) termed current monitoring and evaluation systems weak and noted that there were few sanctions for poor care and little acknowledgment of outstanding care (ABA, 1986). In 1987 the ABA adopted a resolution directed at improving home care quality through the enactment of state and federal legislation and regulation and monitoring systems that focus on the quality of care provided rather than only on the provider's capacity to render care.

Who and what then define the quality of nursing care in the community setting? How has the delicate balance between cost containment and quality of care been addressed? In a rapidly changing environment marked by the explosion of technology in the community setting, the "graying" of the American population, and the general shift in health care delivery from the hospital setting to alternative settings, including home care, how will the nursing profession respond to demands for quality services? These are issues that will remain in the forefront in health policy in the 1990s and beyond.

A REGULATORY APPROACH TO DEFINING QUALITY

Section 1861(o) of the Social Security Act and subsequent Medicare regulations address the Conditions of Participation that a home health agency must meet in order to participate as a Medicare provider of home health services. "Home health agency" under this definition refers to a public or private organization that is primarily engaged in providing skilled nursing and other therapeutic services in the home environment. The regulations and Conditions of Participation address compliance with federal, state, and local laws, organization and administration, acceptance of patients, plan of treatment, medical supervision, skilled nursing, therapy services, medical-social services, home health aide services, clinical records, and evaluation. The responsibilities of the home health registered nurse include conducting the initial evaluation visit; ongoing evaluation of nursing needs; initiation of the plan of treatment and necessary revisions; preventive and rehabilitative nursing procedures; clinical record keeping; coordination of services; communication with the physician, patient, and family; counseling in meeting nursing and related needs; participation in ongoing in-service education; and supervision and teaching of other nursing personnel (Health Care Financing Administration, 1976).

As a result of the Omnibus Budget Reconciliation Act of 1987, the secretary of the Department of Health and Human Services developed and initiated a new home health survey process, which focuses on the quality of services provided to individual beneficiaries, as well as on the quality of care and services the home health agency provides, including home visits to a case-mix stratified sample of patients who are receiving care. This survey process involves unannounced annual reviews by state health department surveyors. The act also added new Conditions of Participation, which address rights of individual patients such as confidentiality, the right to be informed in advance about the care and treatment provided by the agency, the right to voice grievances, the right to have one's property treated with respect, and the right to be informed about the availability of the state home health agency consumer hotline. Additional components of home health aide training also were included in the act (Public Law 100-203, 1987).

ACCREDITATION AS A MARK OF EXCELLENCE

Voluntary accreditation through an on-site peer review, based on evaluation against nationally recognized standards, is yet another approach to the examination of quality in community health nursing. Currently there are three accrediting bodies, including the National HomeCaring Council, the Community Health Accreditation Program of the National League for Nursing, and the Joint Commission on Accreditation of Healthcare Organizations, that offer this mechanism of evaluation.

National HomeCaring Council

The National HomeCaring Council originally established standards that addressed quality in paraprofessional services, such as homemakers and home health aides, as early as 1962. These standards, revised in the years that followed, address four major components in the delivery of home paraprofessional services: structure, staffing, service, and community (National HomeCaring Council, 1981). Structure standards encompass elements such as governance, management, and financial responsibility. Standards that address staffing issues include the provision of adequately trained personnel, personnel practices, and the availability of ongoing staff training. Service standards focus primarily on the referral process, determining eligibility for service, supervision of staff, and case management services. Last, community involvement in the evaluation of the service delivery is addressed in the fourth major component of the standards (Aalberts, 1988). The National HomeCaring Council's accreditation survey is conducted by trained peer reviewers and includes such evaluative mechanisms as policy and procedure review, chart audits, and staff and management interviews.

Community Health Accreditation Program

The National League for Nursing established standards and accreditation for community health nursing programs in 1961, which in 1987 became a fully independent subsidiary known as the Community Health Accreditation Program (CHAP) (Mitchell, 1988). The CHAP accreditation survey is conducted on site annually by trained site visitors who have clinical and management expertise. The survey process begins with a written organizational self-assessment, including an evaluation of community needs and how the organization seeks to address those needs. The on-site review addresses all aspects of the home care organization, including clinical services, financial strength, marketing strategies, human resource capabilities, and strategic planning. Standards specifically address program evaluation, including peer review of the quality of care delivered, as well as client outcomes (Community Health Accreditation Program, 1985).

In its 1986 *Position Statement on Ensuring Quality in Home Health Care,* the board of directors of the National League for Nursing affirmed its belief that it is the responsibility of the nursing profession to establish and uphold standards of home health care. Its report emphasized that the quality of nursing care delivered in patients' homes should be monitored by nurses themselves through a self-regulatory process that relies on nursing expertise (National League for Nursing, 1986).

Joint Commission on Accreditation of Healthcare Organizations

In response to increasing concerns about quality in home care services in the mid-1980s, the Joint Commission on Accreditation of Healthcare Organizations embarked on a 2-year development process to establish comprehensive home care standards that ultimately would address all phases of service delivery to patients/clients in their place of residence. With the guidance of a home care advisory committee composed of representatives from professional associations, trade organizations, consumer groups, and third-party payers, the standards were developed, field tested, and in 1988 published as the *Standards for the Accreditation of Home Care* (Joint Commission, 1988) and revised in 1991 as the *Accreditation Manual for Home Care* (Joint Commission, 1991).

Eligibility criteria for accreditation require that an organization provide directly or through a formal written agreement at least one of the four following services: home health services, personal care/support services, equipment management, and/or pharmaceutical services. These standards include "core" standards that apply to all organizations seeking voluntary accreditation by the Joint Committee: patient/client rights and responsibilities, patient/client care, safety management and infection control, home care record, quality assurance, management and administration, and governing body. In addition, an organization that provides professional nursing services in the home must meet applicable standards in the category "home health services." These standards address the availability, adequacy, and competence of professional staff members and clinical supervision, appropriate communication and coordination with the patient's/client's attending physician, the delivery of services in accordance with initial and ongoing assessments and planned interventions, progress toward the achievement of patient/client goals, drug administration, and the provision of home laboratory services (Joint Commission, 1991).

The on-site accreditation survey is conducted by trained surveyors with advanced educational preparation, as well as a minimum of 5 years of clinical and management experience in the home care field. Evaluation of an organization's degree of compliance with the Joint Commission's home care standards is ascertained through home visits, observation of actual care delivery, interviews with patients/clients, staff and management interviews, policy and procedure review, and home care record review. By mid-1991, more than 2000 home care organizations had successfully achieved Joint Commission accreditation.

The aforementioned three mechanisms of voluntary accreditation offer an organization an avenue beyond minimum licensure or certification that provides expert peer review against nationally recognized standards of optimum care delivery. Organizations that wish to distinguish themselves in a volatile marketplace frequently will pursue accreditation as a demonstrated commitment to excellence in clinical practice. As accreditation evolves to become a standard in the home care field, it is anticipated that consumers and payers increasingly will demand such a mark of quality in choosing a provider of services.

A QUALITY ASSURANCE APPROACH TO CLINICAL EXCELLENCE

An organization's commitment to internal monitoring and evaluation of the quality of services it provides most frequently is demonstrated in its quality assurance program. In all phases of our service industries, the public is demanding proof that an organization sets its own standards of performance and measures its achievement of these standards on an ongoing basis. In the health care arena, one must first evaluate the definition of an assumption surrounding the concept of quality. Donabedian (1987) has described health care quality as the extent to which care provided is expected to achieve the most favorable balance of risks and benefits. From the patient/client perspective, convenience, dignity, and comfort weigh heavily in the definition of quality care. On a broader level, the attributes of quality also might include such components as access to care and equitable distribution of care to individuals of different socioeconomic levels (Donabedian, 1987).

A variety of approaches to the measurement of quality in health care services exists. Assessment of structural components of an organization includes evaluation of staff qualification, adequacy of staffing to meet defined patient/client needs, the existence of clinical and administrative policies and procedures, and the organizational structure that exists (Lalonde, 1987). Donabedian (1986) has noted, however, that this type of evaluation of quality depends on a rather weak and uncertain relationship between the goodness of conditions (structures) and the goodness of care (outcomes). Therefore, although assessment of structures is one component in the evaluation of quality, it should not be the only one. The existence of adequate structures does not in itself guarantee positive outcomes; it merely increases the probability of their realization.

Process assessment refers to what is done in caring for the patient/client, such as the assessment, planning, and intervention component of the nursing process. This approach to quality measurement also is not without criticism. One criticism relates to the reliability of the process, inasmuch as there may be a number of acceptable approaches to an identified patient/client problem or need. Interventions may be carried out that are deemed to be acceptable nursing practice even with little or no research to support the efficacy of the intervention. The validity of process assessments also may be scrutinized, because poor processes actually may have little or no relationship to good quality outcomes (Lalonde, 1987).

Outcome assessment relates to the end product of the care provided—the observable consequences in the patient's/client's physical, social, and/or mental health states (Lalonde, 1987). Increasingly, demands are being placed on health care professionals and organizations to define and measure patient/client clinical outcomes as a component of the organization's evaluation of quality. An example of such an initiative is the Joint Commission's Agenda for Change, a recent research and development endeavor to define clinical outcome indicators in a variety of health care settings and services. Outcome assessment alone, however, cannot tell the entire story about quality. In some cases the best possible interventions may have been provided to the patient/client by qualified and empathetic staff members; because of factors outside the control of practitioners, the health care organization, or the patient/client, the expected outcome may never be achieved by the patient/client (Lalonde, 1987).

JOINT COMMISSION MONITORING AND EVALUATION OF QUALITY AND APPROPRIATENESS

The Joint Commission's home care standards require that "there is an ongoing quality assurance program designed to objectively and systematically monitor and evaluate the quality and appropriateness of patient/client care, resolve identified problems, and pursue opportunities to improve care" (Joint Commission, 1991). Recognizing that the development and maintenance of a meaningful quality assurance program poses a major challenge for home care organizations, the Joint Commission has developed a 10-step model for quality assurance that addresses the major standards in this area. This model may readily be applied to the monitoring and evaluation of community health nursing practice as follows.

Step 1: Assign responsibility. The governing body of the home care organization is ultimately responsible for creating and supporting the organization's quality assurance program. Management and clinical staff members are most likely to be responsible for the actual implementation of the activities. The written quality assurance program should clearly address the delineation of authority and responsibility for all phases of monitoring and evaluation. For example, the patient care coordinator or nursing supervisor may oversee the implementation of the activities, with clinical staff members assuming an active role in data collection, peer review, and analysis.

Step 2: Delineate the scope of care. The home care organization will next want to delineate the scope of services provided, such as professional services or primary clinical activities. Examples of scope of care might include patient/client and/or family education, assessment, drug monitoring, rehabilitative nursing, and maternal/child care.

Step 3: Identify important aspects of care. After the scope of care is described, the next task is to identify those activities that are considered most important to the quality and appropriateness of the care provided. In the evaluation of which clinical activities have the greatest impact on patient/client care, priority should be given to those activities for which one or more of the following services is true:

- The activity occurs frequently or affects large numbers of patients/clients (high volume).
- Patients/clients are at risk of serious consequences or are deprived of substantial benefit if the care or service is not provided correctly, in a timely fashion, or on proper indication (high risk).
- The activity has tended to produce problems for patients/clients and/or nursing staff (problem prone).

Examples of important aspects of care in a community nursing practice are included in the box on p. 126.

Step 4: Identify indicators. An indicator is a well-defined, objective, measurable variable that is used to measure the quality and appropriate-

---

Examples of Important Aspects of Care
in Community Health Nursing

- Education and management of diabetes (high volume, problem prone)
- Management of patients/clients receiving total parenteral nutrition in the home (high risk)
- Wound care (problem prone)
- Education and monitoring of medications for elderly patients/clients (high volume, problem prone)
- Patient/client satisfaction (high volume)
- Pain and symptom management (high volume, high risk, problem prone)
- Management of the patient/client with acquired immunodeficiency syndrome (AIDS) (high risk, problem prone)

---

ness of a defined important aspect of care. Indicators may reflect the structure, process, or outcome of care provided. Authoritative sources for indicator development may be national professional societies, experts in community health nursing practice, or research studies published in recognized professional journals.

Step 5: Establish thresholds for evaluation. Each threshold for evaluation is a preestablished aggregate level of performance (number of clients) that relates to a specific indicator of quality and appropriateness. When the aggregate level of performance reaches the threshold, evaluation is conducted to determine whether a problem or an opportunity to improve care exists.

Step 6: Collect and organize data. Collecting data that describe the actual care provided and a critical analysis of the data are essential elements of the quality assurance process. Some considerations in data collection and analysis include methodology for collection, data sources, individual(s) responsible for data collection and analysis, and the frequency of review. Potential data sources in the community health nursing arena might include clinical records, on-site observation of staff members providing nursing care, incident reports, infection control reports, and patient/client satisfaction surveys. After data have been collected from an appropriate sample size of patients/clients, findings must be compared with the threshold level to identify care or services requiring further review. An example of information for monitoring and evaluating an important aspect of care, diabetes education, is shown in the box on p. 127.

Step 7: Evaluate care. When the threshold for evaluation is reached for a defined indicator, this area should be intensively reviewed to identify problems or areas for improvement. The evaluation might include an

---

_____ **Monitoring and Evaluation of Diabetes Education** _____

Important aspect of care: Diabetes education

Indicator: Before discharge from the home care organization, the patient/client with diabetes or the primary caregiver will be able to verbalize and/or demonstrate correct understanding of diabetes management in the following areas:

1. Diet
2. Medications, including administration of insulin, if applicable
3. Foot care
4. Skin care
5. Use of the home glucose monitoring device
6. Signs and symptoms and appropriate response to hypoglycemia and hyperglycemia

Threshold for evaluation: 95%

Methodology: The nursing quality assurance committee will conduct a review of all patients/clients with diabetes who had been discharged during the previous quarter. Review will occur during the first week of each quarter.

Data source: Clinical records, including diabetes education checklists

---

analysis of trends or patterns related to shifts in personnel, initiation of a new service or patient population, or variations in the skill levels of nursing staff members. The evaluator will want to ask, "Why is this variation occurring, and what can we do to improve performance in this area?"

Step 8: Take action to solve identified problems. Sometimes the evaluation will focus on a particular area of concern such as staff competency, systems difficulties, or staffing shortages. When this occurs, an action plan is formulated to resolve the identified problem or to improve care. Actions might relate to changes in clinical practice, policies and procedures, management practices, or in-service or continuing education.

Step 9: Evaluate effectiveness of actions. After allowing sufficient time for change to occur, a follow-up evaluation is warranted to access the effectiveness of actions taken in resolving identified problems. If the quality and appropriateness do not improve, then the identified problem, its cause, and the action taken to resolve it should be reassessed and new action taken, to be followed once again by evaluation.

Step 10: Communicate relevant information. The organization should use the information gathered through quality assurance activities for internal communication to staff, management, and governing body members, as well as for integrating its findings with other organizations with which it may have a relationship, such as a hospital, clinic, or case manager.

CURRENT INITIATIVES IN QUALITY ASSURANCE

The development and implementation of outcome measurements for the provision of community health nursing have been undertaken by a number of professional organizations and home care providers in recent years. In 1988 the Health Care Financing Administration funded a multi-year study to develop outcome indicators for home health care that in the future may be tied to payment for services.

The Colorado Association of Home Health Agencies (1983) developed outcome audit criteria in 1983 for use in evaluating whether a patient's/client's status is within acceptable ranges. Thirty-six patient care audit nursing topics have been developed, and it is assumed that only one condition exists for each audit. Therefore, if more than one condition exists, multiple audits must be conducted. Examples of topics include chronic intractable pain, wounds/decubitus ulcers, diabetes mellitus, congestive heart failure, and colostomy. For the topic of wounds/decubitus ulcers, outcome criteria address vital signs within normal limits; healed wound or ulcer site; verbalized understanding of treatments, medications, and signs and symptoms of complications; and maintenance of a high-protein, high-carbohydrate, and high–vitamin C diet, among others. Use of outcome audit criteria provides not only for retrospective care evaluation but for concurrent patient care planning and interventions.

The Ramsey County Public Health Nursing Service (Christensen, 1987) has developed and implemented 12 sets of client outcome criteria that are based on criteria developed by the Minnesota Department of Health. These criteria include an evaluation of the patient's/client's knowledge of the situation, the management interventions provided, the extent to which psychosocial adjustments have been made, and the status of discharge. For example, outcome criteria for open wound care include an assessment of the client's understanding of the healing process and the management of the healing process, client's and/or significant others' implementation of the wound management, client's acceptance of necessary life-style adjustment, and wound status. The reviewer evaluates whether the criteria have been met and, if not, explains why they have not been achieved.

The Visiting Nurse Association (VNA) of Omaha has developed a comprehensive quality assurance program that includes three schema or components based on principles of community health nursing practice (Martin & Scheet, 1987). The first scheme, problem classification, represents four domains of practice, including environmental, psychosocial, physiologic, and health-related behaviors. For example, the domain of health-related behaviors addresses such elements as nutrition, sleep and rest patterns, personal hygiene, prescribed medication regimen, technical procedure, physical activity, substance misuse, family planning, and medical/dental supervision. The problem classification scheme assists the community health nurse in categorizing problem areas and referencing them as issues of health promotion, as potential problems, or as deficit/impairment/actual problems. Scheme No. 2 incorporates a problem rating scale of outcomes, which consists of a Likert-type scale that measures the concepts of knowledge, behavior, and status. The ratings are then used as a guide for the community health nurse in planning for patient/client care as evaluations are conducted at periodic time intervals during the course of patient/client care. Scheme No. 3 involves an intervention scheme of nursing activities such as health teaching, treatments and procedures, case management, and surveillance. This scheme is used in conjunction with the problem rating scale as a basis for planning and intervention.

The National League for Nursing's Community Health Accreditation Program (CHAP) has advocated the development and implementation of client outcome program objectives that are measurable, client-oriented goal statements for a defined patient population. Outcomes are recommended in each of three areas: knowledge, behavior, and health status. Examples of an outcome objective in health status might include resolution of an infection, complete rehabilitation, or independence in activities of daily living (ADL). CHAP recommends that the home care organization collect data on an ongoing basis to demonstrate results and to develop a data base for projections of future expected outcomes (Rinke & Wilson, 1988).

The Home Care Association of Washington (Lalonde, 1986), under a federal grant funded by the Health Care Financing Administration, developed and tested a general symptom distress scale for use in evaluation of the patient's/client's response in the home care setting. The scale is intended as a concurrent broad measure of symptom distress across a variety of patient/client diagnostic categories. Symptoms addressed include pain, nausea/vomiting, bowel problems, urinary bladder problems, cough, respiratory problems, swelling/fluid retention, skin problems, speech problems, mood, and activity level. Each symptom is scored on a scale of 1 to 4, providing the health care professional with objective data on the progress, or lack thereof, in managing a patient's/client's distressing symptoms. The general symptom distress score summary can easily be built into an organization's quality assurance program to provide an aggregate evaluation of the organization's success with symptom management. For example, the quality assurance committee could investigate symptoms for which a large proportion of patients/clients reported moderate to severe distress and then aim toward the reduction of the overall incidence of the symptom by the time of the next review (Lalonde, 1987).

As community nursing care has ventured into the provision of complicated technical care in the home, such as management of the ventilator-dependent patient/client, it has been necessary to expand the principles of outcome assessment to encompass this high-risk component of practice. The Visiting Nursing Service (VNS) of Rochester and Monroe County, Inc., has developed and implemented a comprehensive quality assurance program for this patient population, including clinical policies and procedures and outcome criteria for tracheostomy site and cannula care and home care of patients receiving positive pressure ventilation. With use of the outcome criteria format developed by the Colorado Association of Home Health Agencies, the quality of care of the patient receiving positive pressure ventilation can be evaluated by addressing elements such as ventilation equipment maintenance, psychosocial/environmental assessment, and home care process (McC. Votava, Cleveland, & Hiltunen, 1985).

The Joint Commission initiated its first outcome indicator developmental work in home care in the fall of 1990. Outcome indicators under development and field testing are related to the provision of home infusion therapy, which is considered a "high risk" patient service. By 1994, accredited home care organizations that provide home infusion therapy will be required to collect and analyze data comparing their results with those of a nationally recognized data set.

CONCLUSION

As we move through the nineties, community nursing care will continue to hold a significant role in the health care delivery system. Trends toward deinstitutionalization are certain to continue as the population ages and alternative sources of support are sought to maintain elderly persons and those within the community who are chronically ill, terminally ill, or disabled. The consumer movement that began in the decade of the 1960s has stretched into the nineties as well, and nurses in community settings will be asked to demonstrate not only their commitment to quality care but also their success in achieving it. In the home health care arena, significant research studies are currently under way, which will address outcome measurements in patient/client care and in the future most likely will bear some relationship to reimbursement from the federal and state governments, as well as private insurers. Community health nurses must continue to maintain an active role in defining clinical outcomes of quality and in developing and implementing comprehensive internal quality assurance programs, as well as a national data base of outcome measures and findings. With such a proactive posture by the nursing profession, community health nursing will continue to be a key player in shaping health policy into the twenty-first century.

REFERENCES

Aalberts, N. (1988). Homemaker–home health aides: Providing quality services. *Caring*, 7(10), 10-14.

American Bar Association. (1986). The black box of home care quality. A report presented to the chairman of the House Select Committee on Aging, House of Representatives. Washington, DC: U.S. Government Printing Office.

American Bar Association, House of Delegates. (1987). Resolution on home care quality. Resolution approved at annual convention.

Christensen, M. (1987). Development and use of functional client outcomes. In L. Rinke & A. Wilson (Eds.), *Outcomes measures in home care:* Vol. 2. New York: National League for Nursing.

Colorado Association of Home Health Agencies. (1983). *Colorado quality assurance audit criteria.* Englewood, CO: Author.

Community Health Accreditation Program. (1985). *Accreditation criteria, standards, and substantiating evidences.* New York: National League for Nursing.

Donabedian, A. (1986). Criteria and standards for quality assessment and monitoring. *Quality Review Bulletin, 12*(3), 99-108.

Donabedian, A. (1987, January-March). Five essential questions frame the management of quality in health care. *Health Management Quarterly*, pp. 6-7.

Health Care Financing Administration. (1976). Conditions of participation: Home health agencies. *In Medicare and Medicaid Guide.* Chicago: Commerce Clearing House.

Joint Commission on Accreditation of Healthcare Organizations. (1988). *1988 Home care standards for accreditation.* Chicago: Author.

Joint Commission on Accreditation of Healthcare Organizations. (1991). *Accreditation manual for home care:* Vol. 1. Oakbrook Terrace, IL: Author.

Lalonde, B. (1986). Quality assurance manual of the Home Care Association of Washington. Edmonds, WA: Home Care Association of Washington.

Lalonde, B. (1987). The general symptom distress scale: A home care outcome measure. *Quality Review Bulletin, 13*(7), 243-250.

Martin, K. & Scheet, N. (1988). The Omaha system: Providing a framework for assuring quality of home care. *Home Healthcare Nurse, 6*(3), 24-28.

McC. Votava, K., Cleveland, T., & Hiltunen, K. (1985). Home care of the patient dependent on mechanical ventilation: Home care policy development and goal setting using outcome criteria for quality assurance. *Home Healthcare Nurse, 3*(2), 18-25.

Mitchell, M. (1988). The Community Health Accreditation Program: Its strategic meaning to the home care industry. *Caring, 7*(10), 20-24.

National HomeCaring Council. (1981). *Basic national standards.* New York: Author.

National League for Nursing. (1986). *Position statement on ensuring quality in home health care.* New York: Author.

Omnibus Budget Reconciliation Act of 1987, Public Law 100-203, December 22, 1987.

Rinke, L., & Wilson, A. (1988). Client-oriented project objectives. *Caring, 7*(1), 25-29.

CHAPTER 10

Quality in Nursing Home Care

Charlene Harrington

The quality of care provided by nursing homes is of increasing concern as the population ages and the length of stay in acute care facilities declines. Problems encountered with the quality of nursing home care and current government and private efforts to improve quality are discussed in relation to desired client outcomes. Administrators have responsibility for initiating and facilitating structural, personnel, and policy changes that will improve the care provided for nursing home residents.

No issue for nursing homes is as difficult and controversial as quality of care. Of the approximately 19,000 nursing homes in the United States (Hing, 1987) probably more of them offer substandard care than does any other segment of the health care industry. Estimates of the number of nursing homes that operate below minimum acceptable standards vary, but the U.S. Senate Special Committee on Aging (1986) argued that as many as one third are substandard. The U.S. General Accounting Office (U.S. GAO, 1987) conducted a study that found 41% of the skilled nursing and 34% of intermediate care facilities nationally were out of compliance during three consecutive inspections, with one or more requirements considered by experts to be the most likely to affect patient health and safety. Although many nursing homes offer high-quality care, the wide variation in quality indicates the importance of efforts to improve quality of care.

University of California, San Francisco, CA 94143.

Series on Nursing Administration – Volume III, 1992

Variations in quality of care may be related to differences in the management, organization, and financing of nursing home organizations. Discussed here are problems with the quality of nursing home care and the outcomes of care on residents. Current efforts to improve quality of care through the implementation of macrolevel public policies that change the structure, the process, and the outcomes of nursing care are explored. Regulation, reimbursement, accreditation, professional association activities, consumer group activities, and other mechanisms are discussed as important resources to improve quality of care. Nursing home resource management also is basic to reform of quality of care. Management has a responsibility to use all means possible to guarantee not only that minimum standards are met but also that the highest possible quality of care is achieved.

PROBLEMS WITH QUALITY OF CARE

Many studies have described the serious quality of care problems in some nursing homes, which have led to deaths, permanent injury, disability, pain, and discomfort (Pope, Smith, & Romano, 1986; U.S. Congress, 1974-1976; U.S. GAO, 1987; U.S. Senate, 1986; Wood & Pepper, 1988). Since federal fire and life safety regulations were strengthened in the 1970s, most problems with poor nursing home care are directly related to inadequacies in nursing care itself. Problems related to poor nursing care include malnutrition, dehydration, decubitus ulcers, incontinence, infection, overmedication, depression, and other serious physical and emotional problems. Quality of life and residents' rights also are critical components to nursing home care. Frequently cited problems are lack of privacy, lack of consideration for personal tastes, lack of choice about the most basic issues of food and schedules, and discourteous staff members. These common problems have given nursing homes a generally bad reputation with the public, which views these facilities as a place of last resort.

The quality of nursing home care has become a growing concern because residents generally have an increasing level of disability and require increasingly more complex treatments. This change in acuity and dependence has been documented in several studies (Hing, 1987; Shaughnessy, Kramer, & Schlenker, 1987; U.S. GAO, 1983). A number of public policies have encouraged the increasing acuity. The introduction of prospective reimbursement for Medicare-eligible hospital patients has encouraged hospitals to reduce the length of stay and to accelerate discharge (Institute of Health & Aging [IHA], 1985; Neu, 1988). In addition, states are using Medicaid preadmission screening and the home- and community-based waiver programs designed to divert individuals away from nursing homes.

Medicaid case-mix reimbursement systems introduced in some states also have been designed to encourage nursing homes to accept residents with greater nursing care needs (Swan, Harrington, & Grant, 1988). Under these systems, facilities receive higher reimbursement rates for residents with greater acuity levels (Fries & Cooney, 1985). Furthermore, the limited overall nursing home bed supply in some states tends to increase acuity levels (Harrington, Swan, & Grant, 1988; Swan & Harrington, 1986). Bed supply is not expected to meet the growth in demand for care brought about by the rapid increase in the age and disability of the population. The overall increase in demand and acuity levels also can exacerbate quality of care problems.

The quality of care problems and controversies over federal regulation resulted in the Institute of Medicine (IOM, 1986) conducting a 2-year study on nursing home quality of care and regulation. Based on a series of public hearings across the country, a review of the literature, and detailed case studies of selected state regulatory programs, the IOM committee urged immediate federal legislation to improve nursing home regulation and quality of care.

Because of these many problems, Congress passed a major reform of nursing home regulation in 1987, the first significant changes since Medicare and Medicaid were adopted in 1965 (Omnibus Budget Reconciliation Act [OBRA], 1987). Additions and technical amendments to the 1987 legislation have been made annually since that time, and the Health Care Financing Administration (HCFA) has adopted new regulations, procedures, and interpretive guidelines over the past 3 years to implement the legislation. These regulatory efforts have begun a new level of effort to improve nursing home care across the country. This chapter describes many of the regulatory and management changes designed to improve quality of care.

STRUCTURAL CHANGES

Staffing Levels

Although nursing care is the fundamental service offered by facilities, nurses are in short supply (Harrington, 1987). Skilled nursing facilities (SNFs) are now required by federal regulation to have a full-time director of nurses who is an RN and at least one RN on the day shift 7 days a week (OBRA, 1987). During evenings and at night, however, charge nurses may be either RNs or licensed vocational nurses (LVNs). Even though the federal standards require a minimum level of staffing, the regulations require adequate staffing to meet the needs of residents; thus higher staffing levels are compulsory where residents have greater acuity levels. Although many facilities in the country have more professional staff than is mandated by federal regulations, other facilities barely meet or fail to meet the minimum standards.

The most recent national nursing home survey reported 1 RN,

1.5 LPNs, and 6.2 aides per 20 beds (Strahan, 1987). This contrasts with 1 RN for every 4.5 patients in acute care facilities (Aiken, 1981; ANA, 1986). When the number of personnel providing direct patient care is averaged across a 24-hour period 7 days a week, the national average is 1.2 RNs and 8.9 LPNs and aides per 100 residents (Strahan, 1987). One study reported that RNs in hospitals spend an average of 45 minutes in direct nursing care per patient per day compared with less than 12 minutes for RNs in nursing homes (Jones, Bonito, Gower, & Williams, 1987). Thus there are simply too few staff members to provide adequate care to the nation's nursing home residents.

Many of the nation's 1.4 million nursing home residents need complete or partial assistance in bathing, toileting, eating, transferring, and other ADL (Hing, 1987). A large percentage of nursing home residents have such problems as urinary and bowel incontinence, decubitus ulcers, malnutrition, infections, and other conditions that require skilled nursing care. Some homes are now providing intravenous therapy, inhalation therapy, ventilation treatment, and other complex treatments that necessitate RN care. As these demands increase, nursing homes need increasingly professional staff members with special education in gerontology.

Nurses and patients themselves are well aware that quality of care in nursing homes is directly related to the presence of adequate numbers of RNs to assess, plan, implement, and evaluate the care requirements of each patient. The ANA recommends that nursing home staffing be based on a level that ensures the safe and effective delivery of care, addressing the intensity of care needs, the number of hours of nursing care required by patients, and the expertise of the RNs. The ANA has suggested that all nursing homes should have RNs on duty 24 hours a day, 7 days a week, at a minimum, in addition to a full-time director of nursing and a full-time director of in-service education (ANA, 1986).

Limited research suggests a relationship between staffing levels and quality of care. One study in 1977 found a positive relationship between quality of care and the number of RNs (Linn, Curel, & Linn, 1977). More recently, Spector and Takada (1989) found that low levels of staffing in nursing homes in Rhode Island with highly dependent residents were associated with reduced likelihood of resident improvement. High catheter use, a low percentage of residents receiving skin care, and low participation rates in organized activities also were associated with functional decline and death.

More studies on staffing and quality of care in nursing homes are needed. Development of reliable and valid outcome measures for quality of care is needed to facilitate research that will determine the impact of higher levels of staffing on quality of care. Despite the need for further research on quality, improved levels of staffing should receive the highest priority in order to address quality of care problems.

Moreover, public policy makers need to establish higher staffing standards for nursing homes, but the major impediment is the direct costs of such policies on federal and state budgets. Because Medicaid paid some 42% of $55 billion in total estimated nursing home costs in the United States in 1990, it is dramatically affected by any changes in staffing levels mandated by the federal or state government (U.S. Department of Commerce [DOC], 1990). The government is expected to pay for any additional costs of legislation and regulations for the Medicare and Medicaid programs. Public policy makers and public officials face difficult choices in attempting to raise nursing care standards in nursing homes, given the large federal deficit, the large U.S. trade deficit, and growing government health expenditures.

Wages and Benefits

Wages and benefits for nursing personnel in nursing homes are scandalously low. The average RN working in a nursing home earns an annual salary that is 15% to 45% below the salary level of hospital nurses, placing nursing homes at a disadvantage in competing with hospitals and making it difficult for them to recruit and retain nurses. The low wages are exacerbated by the low ceiling imposed by nursing homes on the wages nurses can earn with advanced years of employment. Thus nurses have little incentive to continue long-term employment in nursing homes.

Nursing attendants, who compose 71% of all nursing home personnel, provide the majority of direct care to residents (Strahan, 1987). The attendants deal with difficult working conditions because of staffing shortages and low wages. The wages generally paid to nursing assistants frequently are little more than minimum wage, and often few or no benefits are provided. These low wages, along with the difficult and demanding work required, result in high turnover rates (frequently reported at 100% or more) and problems in recruiting staff.

The American Health Care Association (1988) reported a shortage of nurses in nursing homes; about 60% of the homes had at least one unfilled position. McKibbin (1990) reported that the national vacancy rate for nurses in nursing homes was 19%, which was higher than for any other type of health care facility. As the nursing shortage continues, the problems of poor quality of care will become more acute unless nursing homes are willing and able to raise wages and improve working conditions.

Education and Training

Nursing home personnel have substantially less education than nurses in hospitals. Only 34% of RNs in hospitals, compared with 54% of RNs in nursing homes, are diploma prepared (U.S. Department of Health and Human Services [U.S. DHHS, 1988). Hospital nurses are almost twice as likely to have a baccalaureate degree as are nursing home RNs. The lower level of training is in part related to the wages and benefits paid. Even though few studies have documented the benefits of greater education for nurses, higher levels of education could logically improve the quality of care.

The ANA (1986) recommends that RNs have a baccalaureate degree in nursing and that, in the future, directors of nursing have both experience in long-term care and a master's degree. Moreover, the ANA recommends that all nursing home patients should have access to the services of clinical nurse specialists or nurse practitioners.

The benefits of specialized training have been confirmed in the teaching nursing home demonstration projects (see Small & Walsh, 1988). One study, which compared nursing homes employing geriatric nurse practitioners (GNPs) with matched control homes, found that the use of GNPs resulted in favorable changes for residents (Kane et al., 1989). This study also reported a reduction in hospital admissions and total days in hospitals in those facilities using GNPs. Several other studies have reported that advanced clinical nurse specialists affect quality of care in a number of areas; benefits include reductions in decubiti, use of physical restraints and catheters, incontinence, dependency, psychotropic drug use, enemas and laxatives, emergency room visits, hospital admissions, and infections and falls (Dimond, Johnson, & Hull, 1988; Joel & Johnson, 1988; Mezey, Lynaugh, & Cartier, 1989; Wykle & Kaufmann, 1988). Another recent study (Kayser-Jones, Weiner, & Barbaccia, 1989) found that 48% of hospitalizations could have been avoided if nursing homes had a sufficient number of trained staff members, nurses who could administer and monitor intravenous therapy, and other services such as diagnostic services. Reductions in hospitalization could result in significant cost savings, which could offset the costs of improving the staffing levels in nursing homes.

Recent changes in Medicare reimbursement should encourage the use of nurse practitioners (NPs) and clinical nurse specialists (CNSs) in nursing homes. Medicare now allows for NPs to receive payment for services in nursing homes (OBRA, 1990). NPs, CNSs, and physician assistants (PAs) who are working in collaboration with a physician to supervise the care of residents can certify and recertify the medical necessity for skilled nursing services for Medicare residents (OBRA, 1990). In addition, increases in reimbursement rates paid by Medicare and Medicaid are needed to give NPs and CNSs a greater incentive to work in nursing homes. More important, nursing home administrators must realize the value of such nurse clinicians and increase their employment in nursing homes.

Nursing Assistant Training Requirements

The poor training of nursing assistants also has been a barrier to high quality of care. Before the OBRA legislation of 1987, many of the nursing attendants had little or no training. Only 17 states had mandated training requirements for nursing attendants, and some of the existing training programs were ineffective, especially those in which little formal training was provided and self-certification was allowed (IOM, 1986). State monitoring of training programs has been a problem because of the large number of homes and the lack of state regulatory staff.

The Nursing Home Reform Act (OBRA, 1987) changed the requirements for nursing aide training to address these problems. Since January 1, 1991, nurse's aides must receive, within 4 months of employment, 75 hours of state-approved training and a competency evaluation. Current employees must be evaluated and shown to be competent (OBRA, 1990). Facilities also must provide regular in-service education and performance reviews of all personnel. Implementing regulations developed by the HCFA will specify the detailed requirements for the training and competency evaluations. Thus facilities will be expected not only to provide training but also to ensure that attendants actually are able to deliver appropriate services. In addition, OBRA 1987 required states to establish a registry that includes the names of qualified aides, as well as aides who have neglected, abused, or stolen from residents, and nursing homes are required to check the registry before hiring nursing assistants.

Other Changes

Other structural changes were made under the Nursing Home Reform Act (OBRA, 1987). Nursing home administrators must still be licensed by states, but the law now requires the DHHS to set federal standards for administrators. Facilities with more than 120 beds are required to employ a full-time social worker, and activities directors must be "qualified professionals." Because many nursing homes have not provided social services in the past, it is hoped that this change will begin to meet some of the most pressing needs for social services.

OBRA 1987 also made a number of statutory changes to ensure the rights of nursing home residents. The legislation gave residents' rights a statutory basis. It included the right to establish resident and family councils, to examine state survey reports, and to receive 30 days' notice of transfer or discharge, to appeal a transfer, and to receive relocation assistance. Transfer is permitted only when the resident's welfare or that of others requires it. Ombudsmen, relatives, and visitors are given "immediate access" to residents; agencies that provide health, social, or legal services have "reasonable access." Ombudsmen have the right—consistent with state law and the resident's permission—to examine medical records. In addition, the 1990 OBRA provides that nursing homes must document whether residents have an advance directive (such as a living will or power of attorney) for health care decisions and provide residents with information about state advance directive laws, as well as the facility's policies on such advance directives.

Although OBRA 1987 did not prohibit discrimination against Medicaid recipients in admissions to nursing homes, it did require facilities to maintain identical policies regarding transfer, discharge, and provision of services for Medicaid and private-pay residents. For the first time, OBRA 1987 explicitly forbids duration of stay contracts, third-party guarantors of payment, and solicitation of donations as a condition of admission or continued stay. The law requires facilities to safeguard residents' personal funds.

PROCESS CHANGES

Changes in the processes of nursing home care are expected to be critical for improving the care outcomes for residents. Inadequate resident assessment, care planning, and service delivery have been identified as common problems in the nation's nursing homes (IOM, 1986). Recognizing this need, Congress made resident assessments mandatory in the federal certification requirements under OBRA 1987. Residents' social and medical needs must be assessed upon admission (no later than 14 days after admission) or after any significant change in the resident's physical or mental condition and at least annually. The assessment must use a state instrument and ensure that a minimum data set is collected as specified by the federal government. The assessment must be conducted by an interdisciplinary team and coordinated by an RN who signs and certifies the assessment. Falsification of assessments is subject to civil penalties. The goal of nursing home care mandated by OBRA 1987 is to help residents "attain or maintain the highest practicable physical, mental and psychosocial functioning, in accordance with a written plan of care."

Hawes (Research Triangle Institute, 1988) maintains that resident assessments can be highly beneficial for nursing homes. First, it will help facilities approach assessment and care planning more systematically and improve their range and quality of care. Second, it will provide facilities with information to identify changes in resident status and to modify the care plan. Third, it can be used by facilities to monitor their own performance and enhance the internal quality assurance processes. Finally, Hawes contends that the information generated by the resident assessment system allows the facility to estimate more accurately the need for various resources, such as staffing levels and services, and to improve the planning and evaluating of its allocation of resources.

The assessment instrument, specified as the Minimum Data Set (MDS), was developed by Research Triangle Institute under a contract for the Health Care Financing Administration (HCFA) (Morris et al., 1990). These federal requirements were built on previous research assessments (Katz, Ford, Moskowitz, Jackson, & Jaffe, 1963; Kane, 1981; Kane & Kane, 1987). Resident assessments that comply with the MDS must include identification information (sociodemographic status, living arrangements, payment status, advanced directives, and so forth); customary routine; cognition, communication, hearing, and vision patterns; physical functioning; continence, psychosocial well-being, mood, and behavior patterns; activity pursuit patterns; disease diagnoses, health conditions, oral and nutritional status, oral and dental status, skin condition, medication use, and special treatment and procedures (Morris et al., 1990). Facilities are required to collect a minimum uniform set of data on each resident and to use the data in the care planning process. HCFA eventually will require that some minimum set of data be reported for certification purposes.

HCFA has developed minimum standards for care planning protocols for nursing homes, entitled *resident assessment protocols* (RAPs). The RAPs are triggers and guidelines that can be used to develop a more comprehensive assessment when problems are identified in the use of the RAP instrument and the MDS. The guidelines help in the evaluation of the triggered problems and serve as the basis for the care plan that nursing homes must develop for residents with specific problems. Nurses must assume primary responsibility for the assessment and planning processes, as well as ensure adequate outcomes for patients.

In addition, all facilities are required under OBRA 1987 to have a quality assurance program and committee. The committee must consist of the director of nursing, a physician, and three other staff members. The committee must meet at least quarterly to identify issues and to develop and implement plans of action to solve problems. For example, the facility should examine problems that are unusual, such as the number of resident falls. If these are common, a plan of action for the entire facility should be developed. Regulations can set these requirements, but nursing management personnel must develop the commitment and skill to make quality assurance meaningful.

One area of new regulatory emphasis has been placed on prohibiting nursing homes from using physical or chemical restraints for disciplinary purposes. In order to use restraints, nursing homes are required to show that the use of restraint is needed to treat a resident's medical symptoms or to ensure the safety of the resident and others and must be used only under a physician's order. Nursing homes must conduct a comprehensive assessment to determine the cause of problems and to seek alternatives to the use of restraints. In addition, the use of psychopharmacologic drugs is to be reviewed at least annually.

RESIDENT OUTCOMES

The overall goal of nursing homes is to provide high quality of care to residents. In the past, quality of care has been poorly defined, not only by regulators but also by nursing home managers. The past emphasis of regulatory agencies, since the Medicare and Medicaid programs were enacted, was on structural characteristics and process. The OBRA 1987 legislation mandates monitoring of resident outcome measures in the federal and state regulatory processes. This new emphasis places great attention on resident assessment and planning and on favorable out-comes for patients. What are the outcomes of care that are expected for nursing home residents? These outcomes are easier to specify when a resident is a short-term resident who needs rehabilitation and other services as a means of enabling the individual to return home. For residents with chronic conditions who are not expected to return to the community or their own homes, the outcomes are more difficult to specify. Residents whose conditions include deteriorating medical, func-tional, or mental status require that different types of outcomes be identified and evaluated.

Although technologies are improving rapidly for those who are acutely ill, the ability to define and measure quality of care of nursing home residents with chronic debilitating problems has not been highly success-ful. Nurses now face the ultimate challenge in developing care plans for nursing home residents and measuring and monitoring the outcomes of this care.

Negative outcomes of care are easier to specify than are positive outcomes. Some of the key negative outcomes that generally should be avoided by nursing homes are contractures, decubitus ulcers, dehydra-tion, malnutrition, urinary tract infections, upper respiratory infections, bladder and bowel incontinence, drug interactions, chemical and physi-cal restraints, accidents and falls, pain, and injury. Other negative out-comes such as readmission to the hospital, injury, disability, or death certainly should be examined and prevented if at all possible. Instru-ments can be used to measure the frequency and extent of these prob-lems in individuals and in facilities as a whole. In each instance when a negative outcome develops, the issue is whether such an outcome could reasonably have been prevented or ameliorated with appropriate nursing care. Although individual judgments must be made regarding negative outcomes, protocols can be established to determine whether appropri-ate care and services were provided and to establish whether medical or physical and mental conditions precluded the appropriate delivery of services to each resident.

Positive outcomes of care can be identified by a review of the basic nursing diagnoses and their treatment. To prevent each negative out-come requires the specification of a positive outcome. Because there are no easy answers for defining these outcomes, this task is the ultimate challenge to nursing administrators in nursing homes. If nurse research-ers and clinicians themselves cannot develop outcome measures and goals, then who else will be able do so?

REGULATORY ACTIVITIES

Although nursing homes are required to meet state and federal licens-ing standards, public regulatory efforts have been considered to be seri-ously lacking by most observers (IOM, 1986; U.S. Senate, 1986). State and federal regulations themselves frequently are too vague to be enforceable. In many situations the public sanctions for noncompliance are ineffective because of the complexity of preparing legal actions and the length of time required to enforce such actions. In other situations the administrative enforcement practices are inadequate because of lack of personnel and resources, weak procedures for enforcement, and the reluctance of staff members to initiate sanctions on the facilities.

Lawsuits against the federal government (*Smith v. Heckler,* 747 F.2, 583 [10th Cir.] 1984) and subsequent federal rulings have shown the regulatory process to be inadequate to protect residents. Because of problems with weak regulatory activity at the federal and state levels, the IOM study (1986) recommended reform of the federal Medicare and Medicaid certification procedures. Those reforms passed in OBRA 1987 were the most substantial changes since the Medicare and Medicaid programs were enacted. The new law requires that facilities receive standard surveys at least every 15 months and extended surveys if substandard care is detected. Special surveys may be conducted when there is a change in ownership, administration, or director of nursing. The DHHS is to establish minimum standards for a multidisciplinary state survey team that includes an RN. The federal share of state survey costs increased to 90% in 1991 but will gradually decline to 75% by 1994. HCFA has developed detailed new survey procedures and interpretive guidelines for the regulations.

Both the states and the DHHS are required to employ a variety of new sanctions to bring facilities into compliance, including civil fines, receivership, and closure. The DHHS may continue payments to a substandard facility up to 6 months while the state tries to bring it into compliance, but the state assumes the risk that it will have to repay the funds if the home does not comply.

States must notify ombudsmen, attending physicians, and administrator licensing boards of findings of substandard care. They are required to investigate complaints and to make survey and cost reports and ownership information available to the public. States are required to adjust their Medicaid rates to pay the costs incurred under the law. Rate setting is to be a public procedure. The key question is whether the increase in regulatory activities will have a measurable or visible effect on quality of care in nursing homes. If so, will public policy makers, researchers, and consumer advocates be observing and evaluating such effects?

ACCREDITATION AND ORGANIZATIONAL ACTIVITIES

Accreditation for nursing homes is a voluntary process of review conducted by the Joint Commission on Accreditation of Healthcare Organizations. The accreditation process has established criteria and standards for review and approval by the Joint Commission as an independent body. Unfortunately, these standards are modeled on hospital standards and are heavily weighted toward structure and process measures of care rather than toward resident outcomes. Nevertheless, the extent to which nursing homes seek to meet accreditation standards shows a commitment to quality, indicating that these facilities attempt to go beyond the minimum federal and state regulatory standards. Inasmuch as only a small proportion of facilities are accredited, this is not a process used by most nursing homes.

Professional organization activities of the American Association of Homes for the Aging (primarily with nonprofit members) and the American Health Care Association (primarily with proprietary members) are both important. These organizations have provided extensive educational information, patient care guidelines for assessing quality, and valuable professional meetings. On the other hand, the interests of these organizations are primarily determined by the managers and owners. These associations sometimes take legislative and political positions contrary to those taken by the American Nurses' Association, employee unions, and consumer groups. Regulatory and economic issues are the primary area of dispute among these groups. Unfortunately, the public policy issues are difficult to resolve without consensus across all the interest groups.

Consumer groups, particularly the National Citizens' Coalition for Nursing Home Reform (NCCNHR), have played the most important role in calling quality of care issues to the attention of the general public as well as public policy makers. Through the efforts of NCCNHR and other consumer groups, the IOM 1986 study was commissioned by HCFA. After the report was completed, NCCNHR formed a large coalition of key consumer groups, and the American Nurses' Association and other groups were primarily responsible for the enactment of the OBRA 1987 legislation (NCCNHR, 1988). After the passage of the legislation, the coalition of groups has continued to assist in developing and critiquing HCFA regulations to implement the 1987 legislation. The group also was involved in cleanup amendments that Congress passed in the OBRA 1988 legislation (NCCNHR, 1988). The contributions made by consumer groups working in close cooperation with professional organizations and nursing organizations are invaluable to reform efforts for nursing homes.

RESOURCE ALLOCATION

The nursing home industry is a multibillion dollar business in the United States, characterized by rapid growth in profits and large chain-owned corporations (Harrington, 1984). Nursing homes were a cottage industry until the early 1960s when they began to expand with the infusion of public funds from Medicaid and Medicare. By 1985, 75% of the nursing homes in the United States were proprietary facilities

(Strahan, 1987). A growing number—41% of all nursing homes in 1985—were associated with chains, compared with 28% in 1977. The nursing home industry is consolidating quickly. Blyskal (1981) reported that the 10 largest chains accounted for 10% of the total number of beds in the country, and in 1983, 32 corporations controlled 17% of the beds (LaViolette, 1983). By 1990, the 25 largest nursing home chains managed 378 facilities with 49,570 beds (Rajecki, 1990). Many of the chains are publicly held corporations, and the largest chains (including Beverly Enterprises, ARA Services, and National Medical Enterprises) are listed on the New York Stock Exchange and the American Stock Exchange. Berliner and Regan (1987) reported the continued consolidation of chains and the development of multinational operations.

The health care business is healthy. The price earnings ratios in the nursing home industry were commonly between 14% and 18% from 1978 through 1983 (Moskowitz, 1983). Beverly Enterprises, with $450 million in business in 1982, reported a growth of 700% between 1978 and 1982 (Keppel, 1982). Some states such as California found that the average nursing home facility made a profit of 41% on net equity in 1978-1979 (California Health Facilities Commission, 1981). A similar study in Texas showed an average profit on net equity of 34% for 1978 (Harrington, Wood, Lalonde-Berg, & Bogart, 1983). More recently, some nursing homes have experienced financial losses. Beverly Enterprises reported large losses in 1987. Hillhaven reported a 25% decline in profits in the first 6 months of 1988, and Manor Care also reported a drop in net income in the second quarter of 1988 but a net income increase of 11% for the first 6 months of 1988 (Wagner, 1988). Representatives argue that their declines in profits are largely related to sharp increased labor costs, particularly resulting from the nursing shortage. Chains also invested large amounts of their revenues in capital to acquire other nursing homes during the early 1980s. In 1989, 74% of the 25 largest nursing home chains reported increases in gross revenues, and 95% reported increases in 1990 (Rajecki, 1990).

Nursing homes have made money from their real estate and capital investments through frequent sales arrangements and the use of management lease arrangements to increase revenues. As Vladeck (1980) points out, nursing homes have used the accelerated depreciation policies under Medicare and Medicaid to pay for the capital investments plus their return on equity investments. The complex mechanisms used by nursing homes to increase their profits are difficult to track and to understand for those unfamiliar with the financial arena. Even nonprofit nursing homes operate with a growth imperative, with similar pressures to maximize revenues and control costs. The differences between nonprofit and profit facilities often are blurred and are based on management and distribution of profits rather than on other corporate behavior.

Price increases have continued each year for nursing homes, primarily supported by public dollars. Residents pay for 52% of all bills directly out-of-pocket. Medicare pays only for about 2%, the Veterans Administration and other government sources pay for 4%, and private insurance and philanthropic pay agencies for about 1% of the total care. Because Medicaid pays for 41% of all nursing home costs, state-established Medicaid policies are critical in shaping the industry (U.S. DOC, 1990). Most state Medicaid programs pay nursing homes on a prospective basis by setting ceilings on total facility costs and sometimes on specific cost centers. State Medicaid programs have been adopting policies to reduce the rate increases to nursing homes (Swan et al., 1988). Although nursing homes emphasize their profits and growth to attract potential investors, the industry has argued that higher Medicaid reimbursement rates are needed and has been fairly successful in sustaining its Medicaid payment rates.

In spite of efforts to control costs, overall nursing home cost increases were 11% between 1988 and 1989 (U.S. DOC, 1990). Certainly, nursing wages for those employees in nursing homes have not kept pace with the increases in revenues for nursing homes. Overall, increased revenues appear to have been used primarily for nursing home administration and profits. The IOM Committee (1986) noted that higher reimbursement rates are not sufficient in themselves to improve quality. Unless the increased revenues were used directly for improving patient care, including better wages and working conditions for employees, there is little reason to argue for increased reimbursement to facilities.

There have been many studies and much controversy over the relationship of ownership to quality of care in nursing homes. Several studies have failed to find statistically significant relationships (Kurowski & Breed, 1981; Lee, 1984). On the other hand, other studies have found better quality of care in nonprofit nursing homes (Caswell & Cleverly, 1978; Elwell, 1984; Fottler, Smith, & James, 1981; Gottesman, 1974; Greene & Monahan, 1981). Nursing homes themselves report that governmental and nonprofit facilities have significantly higher staffing levels than do proprietary nursing homes (Strahan, 1987). Hawes and Phillips (1986) showed significant problems with the quality of care as indicated by regulatory violations by chain facilities in Texas. The chains in the study financed their growth by increased allocation of funds to property costs and reduced expenditures on food, staffing, and social services. These chains spent proportionately less than did nonprofit facilities on direct patient care and more on property and administration. Overall, Hawes and Phillips concluded that the research in the field suggests the superiority of nonprofit nursing homes, particularly church-related nonprofit facilities, in delivering quality care.

A critical issue for nursing care is how the financial resources are allocated by the facility. Such resources can be used for profits, for capital needs and expansion, or for personnel or other direct resident care needs. All too often nursing administrators are unaware of their own facility's or chain's financial picture and are not involved in the resource allocation process. The key to ensuring high-quality care has to be one of ensuring adequate financial resources to provide the care.

CONCLUSION

Quality of care in nursing homes is one of the most difficult challenges facing nursing administrators and care providers. Basic structural changes are needed to increase the number of registered nurses and their educational preparation in gerontology. Better training programs and greater numbers of nursing assistants also are needed. Increased wages and benefits and improved working conditions are critical to retaining the current labor force and ensuring high-quality care.

Many improvements in the processes of nursing care are needed. Comprehensive resident assessments by multidisciplinary teams are key to developing meaningful care plans and to improving the delivery of nursing services to residents. More important, nursing care outcomes must be developed and monitored.

New regulatory efforts have been designed at the federal level to reform the standards of nursing home care. The state and federal regulatory process also has been revised under the most sweeping legislation reform since the Medicare and Medicaid programs were adopted. All these efforts are directed toward ensuring that minimum standards are met in the nation's nursing homes. Accreditation bodies, professional organizations, and consumer groups all have important roles to play in improving quality of care.

Probably more important, questions of resource allocations must be faced directly by public policy makers and managers. The evidence shows that wages and benefits have not kept pace with increases in revenues during the 1980s and that chains and proprietary facilities have used their excess revenues and profits primarily for acquisition, capital, and administrative activities. In some facilities and chains, resources need to be reallocated from administration, capital, and acquisition budgets to direct patient care. More public policy attention should be placed on regulation to reduce the trend toward large nursing home chains and regulation of public reimbursement to ensure that increases in reimbursement are used for patient care and other essential services rather than for profits.

REFERENCES

Aiken, L. H. (1981). Nursing priorities for the 1980s: Hospitals and nursing homes. *American Journal of Nursing, 81,* 325-330.

American Health Care Association. (1988). Manpower survey 1987: Preliminary draft report. Washington, DC: Author.

American Nurses' Association, Council on Nursing Administration and Council on Gerontological Nursing. (1986). *Statement on minimal registered nurse staffing in nursing
homes* and *Statement on mandatory training for nursing assistants in nursing homes.*
Kansas City, MO: Author.

Berlinger, H., & Regan, C. (1987). Multinational operations of U.S. for-profit hospital
chains: Trends and implications. *American Journal of Public Health, 77,* 1280-1284.

Blyskal, J. (1981, November 23). Gray gold. *Forbes* 80-81.

California Health Facilities Commission. (1981). *Economic criteria for health planning
report:* Vol. II (FY 1981-82/FY 1982-83, Health Facilities Commission, draft report).
Sacramento, CA: Author.

Caswell, J., & Cleverley, W. (1978). *Final report: Cost analysis of Ohio nursing homes.*
Columbus, OH: Ohio Department of Health.

Dimond, M., Johnson, M., & Hull, D. (1988). The teaching nursing home experiences,
University of Utah College of Nursing and Hillhaven Convalescent Center. In N. Small &
M. Walsh (Eds.), *Teaching nursing homes: The nursing perspective.* Owings Mill, MD:
National Health Publishers.

Elwell, F. (1984). *The effects of ownership on institutional services.* Unpublished manuscript, Murray State University, Department of Sociology and Anthropology, Murray, KY.

Fottler, M. D., Smith, H. L., & James, W. L. (1981). Profits and patient care quality in nursing
homes: Are they compatible? *The Gerontologist, 21,* 532-538.

Fries, B. E., & Cooney, L. M., Jr. (1985). Resource utilization groups: A patient classification
system for long-term care. *Medical Care, 23,* 110-122.

Gottesman, L. E. (1974). Nursing home performance as related to resident traits, ownership, size, and source of payment. *American Journal of Public Health, 64,* 269-276.

Greene, V. L., & Monahan, D. (1981). Structure and operational factors affecting quality of
patient care in nursing homes. *Public Policy, 29,* 339-415.

Harrington, C. (1984). Public policy and the nursing home industry. *International Journal
of Health Services, 14,* 481-490.

Harrington, C. (1987). Nursing home reform: Addressing critical staffing issues. *Nursing
Outlook, 35*(5), 208-209.

Harrington, C., Swan, J. H., & Grant, L. (1988). Nursing home bed capacity in the states,
1978-86. *Health Care Financing Review, 9*(4), 76-100.

Harrington, C., Wood, J., Lalonde-Berg, G., & Bogart, M. (1983). Texas case study: Medicaid, Title XX, and SSI programs. San Francisco, CA: Aging, Health and Policy Center.

Hawes, C., & Phillips, C. D. (1986). The changing structure of the nursing home industry
and the impact of ownership on quality, cost, and access. In G. H. Gray (Ed.), *For-profit
enterprise in health care* (pp. 492-538). Washington, DC: National Academy Press, Institute of Medicine.

Hing, E. (1987). Use of nursing homes by the elderly: Preliminary data from the 1985
National Nursing Home Survey (NCHS advance data from Vital and Health Statistics,
DHHS Publication No. [PHS] 87-1250). Hyattsville, MD: National Center for Health
Statistics.

Institute of Health & Aging and Institute for Health Policy Studies. (1985). *Organizational
and community responses to Medicare policy: Consequences for health and social
services for the elderly.* San Francisco, CA: University of California, San Francisco.

Institute of Medicine, Staff and National Research Council Staff. (1986). *Improving the
quality of care in nursing homes.* Washington, DC: National Academy Press.

Joel, L., & Johnson, J. (1988). Rutgers—The State University of New Jersey and Bergen Pines
County Hospital. In N. Small & M. Walsh (Eds.), *Teaching nursing homes: The nursing
perspective.* Owings Mill, MD: National Health Publishers.

Jones, D., Bonito, G., Gower, S., & Williams, R. (1987). *Analysis of the environment for the
recruitment and retention of registered nurses in nursing homes.* Washington, DC: U.S.
Department of Health and Human Services.

Kane, R. (1981). Assuring quality of care and quality of life in long-term care. *Quality Review Bulletin, 7,* 3-10.

Kane, R., Garrard, J., Skay, C., Radosevich, D., Buchanan, J., McDermott, S., Arnold, S., & Kepferle, L. (1989). Effects of a geriatric nurse practitioner on process and outcome of nursing home care. *American Journal of Public Health, 79,* 1271-1277.

Kane, R. A., & Kane, R. L. (1987). *Long-term care: Principles, programs and policies.* New York: Springer.

Katz, S., Ford, A. B., Moskowitz, R. E., Jackson, B. A., & Jaffe, M. E. (1963). Studies of illness in the aged — The index of ADL: A standardized measure of biological and psychosocial function. *Journal of the American Medical Association, 185,* 914-919.

Kayser-Jones, J., Weiner, C., & Barbaccia, J. (1989). Factors contributing to the hospitalization of nursing home residents. *The Gerontologist, 29,* 502-510.

Keppel, B. (1982). Multihospital affiliation in hand, Beverly aims to double its size. *Modern Healthcare, 12*(6), 70-72.

Kurowski, B., & Breed, L. (1981). *A synthesis of research on client needs assessment and quality assurance programs in long-term care.* Denver: University of Colorado Health Services Research Center.

LaViolette, S. (1983). Nursing home chains scramble for more private-paying patients. *Modern Healthcare, 13*(5), 130-138.

Lee, Y. S. (1984). Nursing homes and quality of health care: The first year of result of an outcome-oriented survey. *Journal of Health and Human Resources Administration,* 7(1), 32-60.

Linn, M. W., Curel, L., & Linn, B. (1977). Patient outcome as a measure of quality of nursing home care. *American Journal of Public Health, 67,* 337-344.

McKibbin, R. C. (1990). *The nursing shortage and the 1990's: Realities and remedies.* Kansas City, MO: American Nurses' Association.

Mezey, M., Lynbaugh, J., & Cartier, M. (1989). Reordering values: The teaching nurse home programs. In M. D. Mezey (Ed.), *Nursing homes and nursing care: Lessons from the teaching nursing homes* (pp. 1-12). New York: Springer.

Morris, J. N., Hawes, C., Fries, B. E., Phillips, C. D., Mor, V., Katz, S., Murphy, K., Drugovich, M. L., & Friedlob, A. S. (1990). Designing the national resident assessment instrument for nursing homes. *The Gerontologist, 30,* 293-307.

Moskowitz, M. (1983, March 28). The health care business is healthy. *San Francisco Chronicle,* p. 50.

National Citizens' Coalition for Nursing Home Reform (1988, March/April). HCFA faces heavy regulatory agenda in Reagan administration's last year. *Quality Care Advocate,* pp. 1-2, 8.

Neu, C. R. (1988). *Posthospital care before and after the Medicare prospective payment system.* Santa Monica, CA: Rand Corp.

Omnibus Budget Reconciliation Act (OBRA) of 1987: Public Law 100-203. Subtitle C: Nursing Home Reform. Washington, DC: Signed by President, December 22, 1987.

Omnibus Budget Reconciliation Act of 1990 (1990). Nursing home reform technical amendments. *Congressional Record, 149.*

Pope, E., Smith, F., & Romano, B. (1986, November 9). California nursing homes: No place to die. *San Jose Mercury News,* pp. 26A-28A.

Rajecki, R. (1990, December). The search for optimum size: 1990 multi-facility operators survey. *Contemporary Long-Term Care,* pp. 26, 28-31.

Research Triangle Institute (RTI). (1988, July 11). Development of resident assessment system and data base for nursing home residents (RTI Technical Proposal No. 213-88-25). Research Triangle Park, NC: Author.

Shaughnessy, P. A., Kramer, P. A., & Schlenker, R. (1987). Preliminary findings from the national long-term care study (Presented to HCFA). Denver: Univesity of Colorado Center for Health Services Research.

Small, N., & Walsh, M. (1988). *Teaching nursing homes: The nursing perspective.* Owings Mill, MD: National Health Publishers.

Spector, W. D., & Takada, H. A. (1989). *Characteristics of nursing homes that affect resident outcomes.* Paper presented at the Gerontological Society of America Annual Meeting, Minneapolis.

Strahan, G. (1987). Nursing home characteristics: Preliminary data from the 1985 nursing home survey (NCHS advance data from *Vital and Health Statistics, 131,* 1-7, DHHS Publication No. [PHS] 87-1250). Hyattsville, MD: National Center for Health Statistics.

Swan, J. H., & Harrington, C. (1986). Estimating undersupply of nursing home beds in states. *Health Services Research, 21*(1), 57-83.

Swan, J. H., Harrington, C., & Grant, L. (1988). State Medicaid reimbursement for nursing homes, 1978-86. *Health Care Financing Review, 9*(3), 33-50.

U.S. Congress, Senate Special Committee on Aging. (1974-1976). *Nursing home care in the United States: Failure in public policy* (An introductory report and supporting papers No. 1-7). Washington, DC: U.S. Government Printing Office.

U.S. Department of Commerce, International Trade Administration. (1990). *Health and medical services: U.S. industrial outlook 1990* (pp. 49-1–46-6). Washington, DC: Author.

U.S. Department of Health and Human Services, Division of Nursing. (1988). *The registered nurse population: Findings from the national sample survey of registered nurses, March, 1988.* Washington, DC: U.S. Government Printing Office.

U.S. General Accounting Office. (1983). *Medicaid and nursing home care: Cost increases and the need for services are creating problems for the states and the elderly.* Washington, DC: U.S. Government Printing Office.

U.S. General Accounting Office. (1987). *Stronger enforcement of nursing home requirements are needed.* Washington, DC: U.S. Government Printing Office.

U.S. Senate, Special Committee on Aging. (1986, May 21). In *Nursing home care: The unfinished agenda:* Vol. 1, p. 2. (Special hearing and report). Washington, DC: U.S. Government Printing Office.

Vladeck, B. C. (1980). *Unloving care: The nursing home tragedy.* New York: Basic Books.

Wagner, L. (1988). Nursing homes buffeted by troubles. *Modern Healthcare, 18*(12), 33-36, 41-42.

Wood, T., & Pepper, M. (1988, May 29-June 5). How safe a haven? (Series of articles). *Kansas City Star.*

Wykle, M., & Kaufman, M. (1988). The teaching nursing home experience: Case Western Reserve University, Frances Payne Bolton School of Nursing and Margaret Wagner House of the Benjamin Rose Institute. In N. Small & M. Walsh (Eds.), *Teaching nursing homes: The nursing perspective.* Owings Mill, MD: National Health Publishers.

Quality in a Changing Environment

The relationship of quality to environmental and professional advances is discussed in the chapters in this section. Each of the chapters, although focusing on a specific environmental aspect, illustrates the fact that change is forcing nurse administrators to develop new areas of knowledge and to become actively involved in the application of new technologies and the solution of current professional problems.

The first two chapters describe the impact of technology on health care quality. The amount of information necessary for patient care and quality assurance continues to proliferate and has created problems with data storage, retrieval, and analysis. In the first chapter, Mowry illustrates how computer technology can provide a viable method of integrating patient data for clinical decision making and quality assurance. In the following chapter, Jacox and Pillar discuss issues associated with increased reliance on technology in health care and the role of the nurse administrator in relation to the use and assessment of technology. The authors outline the relationship of technology and quality, as well as how technology assessment can be structured into quality assurance programs.

The last two chapters deal with issues specific to the nursing profession: (1) the relationship of nursing research and quality assurance and (2) the ensurance of quality in educational programs that prepare nurses for the future. The challenge of integrating nursing research, practice, and quality assurance is the focus of Stetler's chapter. The author recommends and describes the need to develop a broader perspective of research to meet this challenge and addresses the question of research, how it can be used to provide information critical to the question of quality, as well as issues associated with its conduction and utilization.

The final chapter in the series focuses on the educational preparation of nurses and the assurance of quality in educational programs. Molen presents criteria for the evaluation of baccalaureate and higher-degree programs as a framework for the identification of current and potential problems in nursing education and for recommended strategies to combat these problems. The author suggests changes for restructuring nursing education programs. This chapter should be read by all nurse administrators to increase their understanding of the problems faced by nursing education and the role that nurse administrators can have in preparing professional nurses for tomorrow's health care delivery system.

CHAPTER 11

Computerization and Quality

Mychelle M. Mowry

Computerization is providing hospital and nursing executives the data necessary to make management decisions based on optimizing quality while controlling costs. Key to the process is the design of the computerized system, integrated data banks, point of care data entry, on-line medical records, and user-defined "data filters," which will deliver to managers the data necessary to make rapid quality decisions in a considerably constrained fiscal environment.

Our society has progressed from the age of agriculture, via the industrial age, to the information age; likewise, quality improvement (QI) in the health care industry is evolving from an age of peer review, via the criterion age, to the computer age. The purpose of this chapter is to discuss the use of computers in the support of quality nursing care, the impact of computer design to improve data retrieval for quality analysis, and the structure of future quality data banks.

In the midst of a flurry of concern for quality born of cost-containment measures, computers are providing hospital and nursing administrators the means to develop integrated patient-centered data bases that will facilitate quality clinical decision making. Optimizing quality while controlling costs is not impossible. A myth that has arisen in health care is that more money spent is equivalent to better quality. This has seldom, if

Cedars-Sinai Medical Center, 8700 Beverly Boulevard, Los Angeles, CA 90048.

Series on Nursing Administration – Volume III, 1992

ever, been true in most industries, and it is not likely to be true in health care. Optimizing quality, however, requires that all departments in the institution, along with the medical staff, work together to identify inefficiencies in the system, to develop alternative approaches to traditional care, and to implement a logical and effective quality improvement system.

Quality of care is closely tied to each health care provider's and manager's ability to find, assimilate, and process staggering amounts of information. Many quality failures in current systems can be traced to errors of omission that result directly from a failure to discover or to recognize important data at the proper time. An example of the emphasis currently placed on clinical data by consumer groups, buyers of health care, and an increasingly well-informed public is the release in March 1986 by the Health Care Financing Administration (HCFA) of lists of hospitals with mortality rates for Medicare patients significantly higher or lower than the national average. HCFA also released data for nine common medical problems and for surgery death rates by procedure (Wyszewianski, 1988). The lists were intended to help the professional review organizations (PROs) identify hospitals with problems, but, to the consternation of the hospital industry, they were released to the press. Although the data were controversial, the findings were eagerly pursued by consumers.

Computers are playing an increasingly significant role in the pursuit of quality and the efficient transfer of information. Because the acquisition of a computer system is a significant capital investment, several design issues should be carefully evaluated before the choice of a system is made.

DESIGN FOR QUALITY: INTEGRATION

Physicians and hospital and nursing administrators need to recognize the impact of nursing interventions on medical outcomes. Therefore the single most important change that needs to occur in hospital operations — and correspondingly in the design of systems that support efficient operations — is the integration of all clinical data. A major underpinning, therefore, of any automated system in pursuit of quality must be a single, integrated, patient-centered data base. During a patient's hospital stay or clinic visit, voluminous amounts of data from numerous sources need to be correlated and synthesized by providers of care. Each provider will be organizing and processing similar, if not identical, data; however, each will be interpreting the data from a different viewpoint and with a different set of "data filters." For example, data received during the nurse's admission assessment may be critical to the plan of care for the physical therapist, the nutritionist, the social worker, or the discharge planning nurse.

A single data base will ensure that each piece of data is entered only once and is immediately available on-line for all providers of care with appropriate security clearance. Multiple data base systems that are developed by use of "geopolitical" department divisions reduce productivity and decrease effective data exchange and analysis. The need to exchange information among departmental systems should be obvious.

There are two current approaches to developing an integrated data base. One is to purchase a hospital information system (HIS) that has been designed to operate on a single hardware platform (one computer vendor) and a single software platform (applications developed from a single vendor to operate on that specific hardware). Unfortunately most vendors acquire software from multiple sources, attempt to interface the software on a single or even on multiple hardware platforms, and then market it as an "integrated hospital information system." This interfaced product is seldom satisfactory. Different internal data storage organizations and system design views often render the interface awkward and time-consuming. Furthermore, many times data cannot be interchanged at all. Interfaced systems do not support the primary "integrator" of all clinical data — the bedside nurse.

A recent and exciting development in the HIS industry is providing a second approach to accomplishing an integrated hospital data base. A concept termed *open systems architecture* is being actively pursued by many health care organizations. Vendors are beginning to develop connectivity software that recognizes and supports this new processing environment. An open architecture system involves the use of multiple applications, typically from different vendors, usually on separate computers. These systems are connected through a local area network (LAN). Data are then sent among such diverse systems as laboratory, pharmacy, admitting, and nursing to create an integrated hospital data base. It is an "open" architecture because standard communication protocols — such as health level seven (HL7), or MEDIX (IEEE 1157) and MIB (IEEE 1073) — are used to allow the various systems to "talk to each other." A centralized repository, the integrated hospital data base of selected clinical and management data, is created and available for consolidated presentation and analysis. The computers work intimately together on the network, essentially creating the environment of a single machine through cooperative processing. What makes this possible are new mainframe-caliber microprocessor chips (megachips) and superservers (computers with enormously large disk-drives). These new systems will reside on industry standard networks such as Ethernet. The primary standard in this scenario is not a particular vendor or make or model of computer. Rather, the standard is adherence to "open" or industry-wide standards for communication and data exchange. This technology was developed in the eighties and is now widely used outside the health care industry.

Providers of care should have access to a unified view of all patient information in order to schedule and plan care and to monitor the care delivery process and patient outcomes. An example is instructive: an oncologist attempting to order a chemotherapeutic drug such as bleomycin should first consider the therapeutic value relative to the patient's recent white blood cell and platelet counts and should order the dosage in relation to the patient's body surface area (height and weight calculated). Further, the nurse should consider a periodic respiratory assessment because of the medication's caustic respiratory side effects. The order entry system should automatically display all pertinent information on a single screen — laboratory data, height and weight data (acquired from the nurse's admission assessment) — to facilitate a rapid and accurate clinical decision by the physician (Fig. 11-1). The system also should "suggest" a respiratory assessment for the nurse once the order is placed (Fig. 11-2). This type of data integration and display has obvious cost, productivity, and quality implications that will be discussed later.

DESIGN FOR QUALITY: DATA REVIEW

The quality and quantity of data required to monitor and evaluate the patient care process in a cost-constrained environment ultimately will mandate a virtually paperless system. In the years ahead, the entire medical record will be automated and available on-line.

As the volume of data on-line increases, the need for "critical filters" increases. Humans are extremely well qualified to deal with exceptions, to set goals, to establish priorities, and to perceive relationships. Humans, however, are poorly suited to deal with repetition and to retain both accuracy and speed with data collection and analysis. Computers and humans have complementary sets of attributes, as shown in Fig. 11-3. The ideal design for data presentation and analysis is to build on the strengths of people and computers and to diminish the weaknesses.

The appropriate synergy between computer and human is best demonstrated by systems in which the computer examines all data against a set of human-defined criteria and presents exceptions for human review. All data should be available on-line; however, the computer should segregate data into nonexceptional and exceptional categories for each individual user or each class of users. The goal is to enhance the user's ability to manage large amounts of information effectively.

Myriad factors are in place today to discourage quality nursing care. The nursing shortage, a larger number of higher acuity patients, shorter lengths of stay, and cost containment are but a few of these factors. Nurses are responsible for a greater number of sicker patients and often have less support from ancillary personnel. In this type of environment an abnormal finding can easily be overlooked or delays can occur in the transfer of important information from nurse to physician. A properly designed computer system should automatically highlight abnormalities and route them to all appropriate providers of care. The system should

Phone by Jeter,Harry T,Jr. at 25 Mar 88 1323   Fri, 25 Mar 88   1318

Location	Current Loc	Name	Visit Number	Sec	Age	Physician
4028	IN 4028	Christie,Agatha	1654866-02	F	83Y	Jeter,H

Bleomycin Sulfate New Order

Current Clinical Values

** White Count	16	** Creatinine	0.4
** Platelets	200	** BUN	20
** Hematocrit	35	** Pulse	88 bpm
** pH	7.40	** BP	150/88 mmHg
		** Temperature	99.2 F (37.3 C)

** Body Surface Area   1.3665 M2

Dose

11 Dose (U/M2)	10 U/M2	12 Dose (Units) 14 units
13 When	Friday, 25 Mar 88 1323	
14 DC Time	Indefinite	
15 Comments		

Select number to edit

FIG 11-1 Order entry system display. (From Health Data Sciences Corporation, San Bernadino, CA. Used with permission.)

Phone by Jeter,Harry T,Jr. at 25 Mar 88 1323

Fri, 25 Mar 88 1318

Location	Current Loc	Name	Visit Number	Sec	Age	Physician
4028	IN 4028	Christie,Agatha	1654866-02	F	83Y	Jeter,H

Bleomycin Sulfate New Order

Procedure

                                  Complete
                          Status   MD Nurse
(1) Beleomycin Sulfate always order yes yes
     10 U/M2 25 Mar 1323

(***) Ventilation Assessment always order yes yes
       qd x3

Order procedure(s) with current parameters?   y

FIG 11-2 Order entry with procedure suggestion display. (From Health Data Sciences Corporation, San Bernadino, CA. Used with permission.)

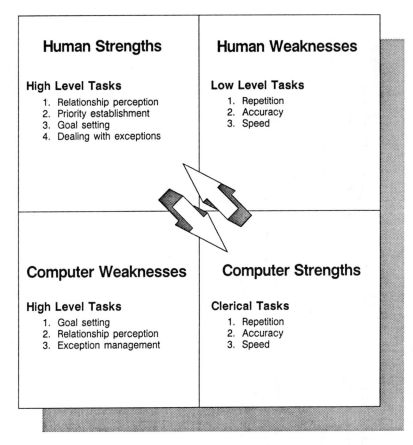

Human Strengths

High Level Tasks
1. Relationship perception
2. Priority establishment
3. Goal setting
4. Dealing with exceptions

Human Weaknesses

Low Level Tasks
1. Repetition
2. Accuracy
3. Speed

Computer Weaknesses

High Level Tasks
1. Goal setting
2. Relationship perception
3. Exception management

Computer Strengths

Clerical Tasks
1. Repetition
2. Accuracy
3. Speed

FIG 11-3 Complementary strengths and weaknesses of computers and humans. (Reprinted from *Managing Health Care Costs, Quality, and Technology,* by M. M. Mowry and R. A. Korpman, p. 171, with permission of Aspen Publishers, Inc., © 1986.)

have the ability to route any type of data, whether from a nurse's assessment, a laboratory finding, or a physician's progress note (Fig. 11-4).

DESIGN FOR QUALITY: DATA MANIPULATION

An automated quality assurance system that is properly designed should provide nurse managers with a review mechanism that replaces group accountability at the unit level with individual accountability and tracks the nursing process for individual patients while concurrently evaluating these activities according to a set of previously defined standards. Nurse managers are ultimately responsible for the quality of care rendered to patients on their units. Individual professional accountability tracked for individual patients is accomplished when a time, date, and signature stamp is attached to all documentation. The manager then is

```
Phone by Jeter,Harry T,Jr. at 25 Mar 88  1323                          Fri, 25 Mar 88   1318

  Location      Current Loc   Name            Visit Number   Sec  Age  Physician
  4028          IN 4028       Christie,Agatha  1654866-02     F   83Y  Jeter,H

     Date                     Procedure             Type           STAT  Abnorm
( 1) Thu, 24 Mar 88   Time    Seizure Assessment    review order
( 2)                  1257    Barium Enema          review order
( 3)                  1235    Transfer              review results
( 4)                  1115    Shift Assessment      review results       yes
( 5)                  0906    Discomfort Assessment review results       yes
( 6)                  0535    Complete Blood Count  review order
( 7) Wed, 23 Mar 88   2000    Progress Note         review results


                              Select event(s) to review
```

FIG 11-4 On-line Review Queue highlights abnormalities and action items. (From Health Data Sciences Corporation, San Bernardino, CA. Used with permission.)

able to review documentation by patient or patient type, by provider, and by medical or nursing diagnosis. Nursing information systems are young and dynamic, however, and nursing standards, which can vary with patient age, diagnosis, and comorbidities, are not yet well-defined. Standard nursing interventions are constantly changed as computers shorten the time required for the dissemination of new knowledge. The process of tracking nursing interventions according to set standards, therefore, requires a flexible automated system that can be adapted to keep pace with new knowledge.

Nurses, as well as other professionals, should be able to alter the data base to adjust to the dynamic nature of their practice. Further, they should be able to require documentation that depends on the nature of the clinical situation or intervention, or both. This process allows clinicians to "force" compliance to previously agreed upon standards. For example, a nursing standards or QI committee can decide that when nurses document a patient seizure, they will be automatically routed through several other data elements or "required fields" such as vital signs, side rails up, description of seizure activity, and notification of physician. Nurses must then fill these required fields before they are able to place their electronic signature on the documentation (Fig. 11-5).

Many quality enhancements are possible when data base development and ongoing modifications are placed in the hands of clinical professionals as opposed to data processing professionals. Further, the ability to require data entry, to route exceptional data, and to modify programs as new knowledge dictates offers a quality control mechanism that has not been previously available.

DESIGN FOR QUALITY: POINT OF CARE DATA ENTRY

The overwhelming interest in bedside-based computer systems is evidence that data documented at the source of data generation (point of care) are more efficient for the provider. People will more readily change and adjust to things that make their lives easier. The data required for health care documentation are generated by patients who typically are located either in a bed or in an ancillary department or clinic, not at a nursing station. Most existing patient care systems, however, have been located at the nurse's station, thus encouraging the archaic process of gathering data at the bedside, holding it in memory (human, that is!) or transferring it from form to form, and at some later time entering it in a medical record kept at the nurse's station. The simple process of moving data documentation to the bedside has quality implications even in manual formats. Whenever providers of care are required to document in multiple places or the environment encourages "memory logs," the possibility of errors and omissions in documentation is increased.

An automated system should provide a tracking mechanism for all

```
Location    Current Loc    Name                Visit Number    Sec  Age  Physician

4028        IN 4028        Christie,Agatha     1654866-02      F    83Y  Jeter,H

                           Seizure Assessment

New Event Time    Fri, 25 Mar 88    0104    Prev Event Status    (unscheduled)

Seizure                                      L clonic contr(jerking) and incontinent urine onset
1  Motor Activity                            without warning duration: 1 min
2  Seizure Description                       lethargic-sleeps often, responds slowly/appropriately
3  Level of Consciousness                    disoriented to person, place & time intermittently
4  Orientation
5  Skin Description                          Blood Pressure: 110/74 mmHg Description: L arm ...
6  Blood Pressure                            Pulse Rate: 68 bpm Description: left radial regular
7  Pulse                                     Rate: 14 bpm Description: normal Effort: unlabored
8  Respirations
9  Physician Notification
10 Safety Precautions


Select number to edit or Choose to mark (M)
```

FIG 11-5 Computer system display showing required documentation. Underlining automatically routes data to Clinicians Review Queue. (From Health Data Sciences Corporation, San Bernadino, CA. Used with permission.)

nursing and physician orders in a format that is automatically updated anytime an order is entered or a care plan is developed. Such a tracking system should be a chronologic schedule of all activities required for an individual patient (Fig. 11-6). Nurses can then access this schedule at the point of care to determine not only those interventions they need to perform but also all activities to be provided by other caregivers. Nurses are the ultimate "integrators" for patient care. It is the bedside nurse who determines after a patient has received medications and suctioning and has been positioned for sleep that the intermittent positive-pressure breathing treatment could be postponed while the patient receives some much-needed rest.

Appropriate interventions also should be tracked through the order entry process. For example, an order placed for a barium enema should automatically schedule all the appropriate associated procedures related to the test. On the evening before the examination the patient's schedule would reveal a need for cleansing enemas, medications such as castor oil (Neoloid), diet changes, and so forth. Numerous associated procedures must be performed in lock step if the examination the next morning is to be successful. In most institutions, however, large numbers of radiologic examinations must be repeated because of inadequate patient preparation. The ramifications for both cost and quality are obvious.

The nursing shortage coupled with more dependent patients requires automated systems that can track every order, intervention, and observation. These activities need to be documented and available at the point of care and highlighted for providers whenever activities are late or when immediate action needs to be taken. An integrated, point of care system will significantly reduce errors that result in major quality failures. The majority of quality indicators and criteria are related to the timeliness and completeness of documentation, both of which are positively affected by bedside-based data entry systems.

QUALITY SYSTEMS ACTUALIZED: FUTURE DATA BANKS

Once a system has been appropriately designed to encourage and support on-line quality measures, it is then up to nursing administrators, physicians, and ancillary administrators to evaluate the data and to implement corrective procedures. Through this quality assurance effort, care is then studied and revised at the department, unit, and individual levels to determine whether the desired patient outcome was achieved in the most productive manner by the time of hospital discharge. To accomplish this goal, an assessment of the adequacy of care is made by reviewing outcomes, content, processes, resource use, and efficiency. Typically, criteria are established against which the desired quality of care and standard of productivity can be measured. These criteria should cover structural, process, and outcome standards.

```
                                                          Fri, 25 Mar 88   1318

Location    Current Loc    Name              Visit Number    Sec  Age  Physician

4028        IN 4028        Christie,Agatha   1654866-02       F   83Y  Jeter,H

(  ) 1) 1600 IV :Cefoxitin        (  ) 11)          ASM:Shift Asm        (  ) 21) brk  NTR:Low Sodium
(  ) 2)      ASM:BwlElim Asm      (  ) 12)          ACT:BR w/BRP         (  ) 22) 0800 IV :Cefoxitin
(  ) 3) 1635 ASM:Vital Signs      (  ) 13)          HYG:Mouth Care       (  ) 23)      ASM:BwlElim Asm
(  ) 4) sup  NTR:Low Sodium       (***)             Fri, 25 Mar 88       (  ) 24) 0835 ASM:Vital Signs
(  ) 5) 1800 MED:Aldomet          (  ) 15) 0000 IV :Cefoxitin            (  ) 25) am   NTR:I&O
(  ) 6) 2000 IV :Cefoxitin        (  ) 16)          ASM:BwlElim Asm      (  ) 26)      NTR:Weigh Pt
(  ) 7)      ASM:BwlElim Asm      (  ) 17) 0035 ASM:Vital Signs          (  ) 27)      ASM:Shift Asm
(  ) 8) 2035 ASM:Vital Signs      (  ) 18) 0400 IV :Cefoxitin            (  ) 28)      ACT:BR w/BRP
(  ) 9) 2200 MED:Aldomet          (  ) 19)          ASM:BwlElim Asm      (  ) 29)      HYG:Mouth Care
(  ) 10) noc NTR:I&O              (  ) 20) 0435 ASM:Vital Signs          (  ) 30) day  LAB:UA


Patient Care Options

( C) Specimen Collection        ( M) Medication Admin        ( T) Shift Summary
( E) Product Ordering           ( O) Order Entry             ( U) Unscheduled Procedures
( F) Face Sheet                 ( P) Care Planning           ( V) Chart Review
( K) Patient Kardex             ( Q) Review Queues           ( W) Work Queue


Select event(s) or Select patient care option
```

FIG 11-6 An automated, chronological patient care schedule. A by-product of Order Entry and the Care Planning Process. (From Health Data Sciences Corporation, San Bernadino, CA. Used with permission.)

Structure

The structure domain encompasses the setting, instrumentalities, and conditions where and under which the provider-client relationship occurs. Structural standards are the foundation of all other standards and define the set of conditions and mechanisms basic to the provision of care. The computer system discussed herein is an integral part of the structural component of quality monitoring. The following are examples of structural issues and how they would be addressed within such a system.

Nurses frequently transport patients who do not require observation simply because it is easier to do it themselves than it is to notify transport services. The automated system should notify transporters on-line by means of a departmental "work queue" function whenever an order is placed for a transfer or a diagnostic examination. Transporters logging on and off the system each time they reach a destination will be notified immediately of any new orders. Nurses should not have to telephone or "beep" for such services. Statistics can be easily obtained to determine response time between transfer order and patient pickup, as well as between pickup and drop-off. These reports may be generated for individual transporters or for department and destination. Performance appraisals would become more objective, patient services would be expedited, and even identification of poorly functioning elevators might facilitate appropriate corrective measures.

Nurses frequently move back and forth between patient rooms and supply rooms. Placement of a terminal in the supply room will allow nurses to identify treatments for several patients at one time, to gather the necessary supplies, and to avoid much unnecessary travel. Nurses are also frequently telephoning and "running down" to central supply because a tray for lumbar puncture was "never sent up!" Terminals placed in central supply with a department or individual (whichever is appropriate) work queue allow for the immediate and automatic transmission of needed supplies when an order is placed in the system.

Studies of activities performed by nursing staff members have shown that 35% to 55% of nursing time is spent in clerically related and other nondirect patient care activities (Mowry & Korpman, 1986). In addition to this voluminous clinical record keeping, nurses often prepare requisitions, maintain unit supply inventories, perform filing duties, and maintain bed census. These activities may be totally eliminated or at the very least significantly decreased with a properly designed computer system. When all documentation is on-line, there is no need for requisitions because orders are transmitted by the system, supply records become a by-product of the on-line documentation process, as does bed census. The data are updated in real time and thus become much more accurate. Further, data are available wherever terminals are located, which eliminates the need to hunt for charts or send a nursing supervisor to locate an old medical record.

Other examples of structural standards involve the staff quantity, level, and quality, all of which may be directly affected by a good computer system. When all treatments and procedures, including the nursing care plan orders, are recorded on-line, it is possible to accurately determine patient needs and thus staffing and assignment data. Because real-cost data are necessary for developing maximally efficient and effective quality patient care plans, a standard and an accurate method for measuring variable nursing resource costs from patient to patient over the entire length of stay is needed. It is difficult to maximize quality and minimize waste without precise knowledge of the time and costs involved in providing care. Obtaining actual nursing cost data by DRGs allows legitimate comparison of nursing with other departments, permitting allocation to nursing of the appropriate portion of increasingly scarce revenues.

When terminals are located at the point of care, it is possible to time all direct patient care activities either ongoing or periodically in order to update standards. It is also possible to update patient status (acuity level) according to new orders or nursing problems. New modalities of staffing will be developed as statistical reports compare patient outcomes with staffing levels, staffing mix, and individual nurses' experience and education (all in-service and personnel records should be kept on-line).

These are but a few of the structural processes that are affected by a properly designed computer system. A system designed to optimize operations will inherently improve the quality of care being given by the users.

Process

The process domain focuses on the activities, pursuits, and behaviors of nurses. These include all that they do or do not do in the course of delivering care. A classic work by Aydelotte and Tener in 1960 could not demonstrate a significant relationship between nursing activity and patient welfare and between in-service education and patient welfare. More than likely, this stems from the nature of nurses' work and the antiquated processes available for nursing documentation. Nurses often address subtle behavioral, psychosocial, or cognitive problems that are rarely documented in manual or even nursing station–based automated systems. Further, numerous providers have an impact on patients during their hospitalization. Therefore there may be overlap with process and outcome criteria of other health professionals. The nursing profession is far from completing a quantifiable list of nursing diagnoses or problems with which goals, interventions, and outcome criteria may be established. These issues have made process quality improvement difficult and have encouraged departmental audits as opposed to integrated patient-centered audits.

Procedures, protocols, standards, guidelines, standards of care, and standard care plans are typical approaches used in addressing process quality improvement. Procedures usually are kept in a notebook somewhere on the unit and provide specific details of how to perform various nursing interventions, for example, how to insert a Foley catheter or how to assist with a bronchoscopy. Procedures need to be updated frequently to keep pace with changing technologies and to meet current performance criteria. When the procedure manual needs updating, there typically is a flurry of activity around the photocopy machine and at least one person spends a significant amount of time on every unit exchanging old pages for new pages. The time and expense involved in this process are only two of three reasons for "computerizing" the procedural change. When a nurse or a nursing student needs a quick reference, it is needed at the patient's bedside. While the equipment for a procedure is being set up, why not have the ability to call up the appropriate screen on the terminal in the patient's room? Furthermore, think how much human resource would be saved if the procedure manual could be updated by an individual on-line in his or her office and made immediately available to everyone throughout the hospital.

Protocols or practice guidelines are plans for treatment written to specifically define what is to be done for a certain category of patients. Newer systems designed to accommodate extensive data manipulation by the customer allow clinicians to alter screens, assessments, protocols, and basically their entire documentation process without ever engaging the vendor. Protocols and practice guidelines for every nursing diagnosis or procedure may then be developed and maintained for each admitting medical diagnosis. As discussed previously with the barium enema example, orders may have associated procedures that reflect protocols or guidelines. The administration of magnesium sulfate to a patient with toxemia exemplifies the usefulness of a computer to coordinate and schedule activities and to notify numerous departments in order to avoid quality failures. The following procedures might automatically be ordered (after physician and nursing approval) and scheduled to be performed—thus appearing on the patient care schedule—when the medication is ordered by the attending physician:

1. Patient education regarding procedure and possible effects
2. Bed rest and quiet room
3. Side rails up
4. Emergency toxemia tray
5. Fetal monitor
6. Vital signs every hour
7. Patellar reflexes check every 4 hours
8. Intake and output (I&O) every hour or every 4 hours in the absence of Foley catheter
9. Magnesium levels
10. Toxemia assessment

These 10 items are included in the usual process quality criteria for the administration of magnesium sulfate. Physicians, nurses (on more than one shift), and phlebotomists must coordinate these activities to ensure proper care of the patient. The automated patient care schedule (Fig. 11-6) should be designed to be used by all providers throughout the patient's day. It should be automatically updated with each order or care plan change. When procedures have been documented, changes in the screen should differentiate them from procedures to be performed. The next activity to be performed should be obvious to the user, and the schedule should move dynamically throughout the day. An on-line integrated schedule then becomes the working tool for providers at the bedside. Any procedure that has been missed should be highlighted for the nurse. Integrated lists of all patients assigned to a nurse and the interventions ordered should be available so that all providers of care can be assured that they have completed everything that should be done for each patient.

This same function (patient care schedule), as well as required fields in the actual documentation process, ensures that standards are being followed. Standards may be general, such as the following:

1. Seventy-five percent of all pain medication will be followed by documented effectiveness on the medication administration record.
2. All patients will be classified correctly.
3. All patients will have assessments on admission and every shift.
4. An I&O record of all patients with intravenous (IV) lines will be maintained.
5. There will be an individualized care plan for each patient.

Each of these standards could be expeditiously handled in the automated environment in the following manner:

1. Each pain medication administered would automatically generate an "associated procedure" that would appear on the patient care schedule one-half hour after the pain medication is given. This simple assessment would require the nurse to document medication effect. Seventy-five percent compliance is hardly appropriate for those who happen to fall in the 25% category. With this system there would be no reason not to expect 100% compliance.
2. The system would automatically classify patients according to physician orders and nursing orders (by means of the care planning processor). These data would be automatically calculated for the staffing coordinator.
3. Each unit would have the ability to "predefine" its "unit orders." Thus, when the patient is admitted to the unit, an admission assessment would appear automatically on the patient care schedule, as well as an assessment for each shift. These assessments are de-

signed by unit and may contain standards of care that become required fields to be documented for each patient.
4. The order for I&O maintenance would be automatically generated when a physician orders IV infusions for the patient. Each time an IV line is changed or a Foley catheter emptied, the nurse would document the volume at the bedside, and the system would automatically update the I&O record. Thus the record would be always up-to-date, accurate, and available to all who need to know.
5. The system would prompt the nurse at each step of the nursing process. It would suggest a nursing diagnosis after scanning the assessments performed on each individual patient for the previous 24-hour period.

Standards also may be specific to the patient and the nursing diagnosis. The Joint Commission on Accreditation of Healthcare Organizations is requiring very specific criteria and discharge plans for each nursing problem defined (O'Leary, 1987). Myriad process variables will be affected by computerization in the years ahead. Properly designed systems should encourage single accountability and concurrent review by unit managers.

Outcome

The final and most difficult aspect of a quality model is the outcome domain. Several problems have been apparent over the years: (1) it cannot be assumed that measured change is the direct result of goal-directed nursing care; (2) the development of a set of measurable outcome criteria specific to nursing is in its infancy; and (3) work has barely begun on developing reliable and valid methods of measuring outcomes. These problems are further exacerbated by the unreliability of nurses in documenting care plans and their related activities.

The following are typical criteria related to care planning:

1. A care plan will be started within 24 hours of admission.
2. The identified care plan interventions are documented in the chart.
3. The care plan reflects updating/revision.
4. The care plan addresses individualized patient needs.
5. Outcome goals will reflect discharge planning.

Again, a properly designed system will significantly affect adherence to the aforementioned criteria and, further, will address the perennial problems that occur in measuring outcomes.

Care planning in a manual system or even most automated systems to date is difficult. Nurses typically are given a blank Kardex on which to develop the plan of care for each patient or, at best, are handed a "standard care plan" that is to be "personalized" and "individualized" for each patient. Short of a dissertation on our present nursing educational process, note at least the gap between the manner in which nurses are educated to write care plans and the reality of what is possible in the day-to-day working world. Nurses should have a prompting process to guide them through the care planning exercise for each patient. Further, they should be reminded to update and revise the plans of care. The care planning process begins with the admission assessment, which should be automatically scheduled for each newly admitted patient, thus appearing on his or her "patient care schedule." The actual process of care plan development should be automated and available at the bedside so that it becomes very natural for the nurse to complete the plan of care after interviewing and assessing the patient.

A list of possible nursing diagnoses should be "suggested" by the system after it evaluates the exceptional data entered during the admission assessment. Nurses may then choose to develop one of the suggested diagnoses or to select from a list of acceptable diagnoses. They should then be presented with the definition and defining characteristics of the diagnosis selected. The next screen should prompt nurses to select measurable goals that may be altered for each patient. The process of prompting continues as nurses are guided through appropriate orders and time determinations for reevaluating their interventions. The entire process is documented on-line, giving nurse managers the ability to concurrently review care plans from a terminal or work station in their office and to request an incomplete work list on-line that will highlight an individual's failure to comply with standards.

The nursing orders should be handled in the same manner as physician orders so that they appear on the patient care schedule and are highlighted if they are late or missed entirely. Each nursing order should be accompanied by a result profile that requires on-line result documentation. The system should automatically remind nurses to update the plan of care according to standards or professional decision. Each time an assessment is documented, the patient-specific exceptional data should update the "suggested" diagnoses list. Discharge plans should be listed with the appropriate nursing interventions by diagnosis.

The greatest obstacle in the outcome domain for nursing is the lack of solid research to verify what nursing is contributing to patient progress. Without having the entire nursing process on-line, it is almost impossible to gather data, to determine what nursing is doing and how often, and to know whether it is appropriate. Future data banks will significantly enhance the quality of research directed toward and the development of measurable outcome criteria and valid and reliable measuring tools that are specific to nursing.

CONCLUSION: THE FUTURE IS NOW

Enhanced communication through rapid and accurate data retrieval and analysis is mandatory for adequate quality review mechanisms. The single largest stumbling block in quality enhancement faced by nursing administrators is the inability to pull together all the data in the medical record in a rapid and logical fashion and to be assured that the information is complete and accurate. Pieces of information reach various committees or providers, but all the data relevant to quality never get to all committees and providers in a timely manner. Most of the significant information recorded on a patient is lost to follow-up because of arcane methods of documentation. If data were available quickly and accurately for all providers, the enhancement in quality and the reduction of cost from duplication, errors, and decreased length of stay would be impressive.

Rapid and accurate data retrieval and analysis are made possible with the aid of technology that is available today. An integrated, bedside-based (point of care) system provides concurrent review of all activities, tests, medications, procedures, and plans of care for a patient. When a manual system is automated, it should result in a better system and should optimize operations. Automated systems that basically mirror the manual system promote all the transcription errors, approximations, redundancies, and omissions inherent in manual operations. The quality and quantity of data required to monitor care mandate a virtually paperless system. The entire medical record will be automated and available on-line in the years ahead.

Concurrent quality assurance similar to that used in the automation of large industries will proliferate in the hospital industry. This process requires quality assurance throughout the production cycle. The design concepts discussed for a hospital information system parallel exactly the innovations being adapted by firms in other competitive environments. Should consumers settle for less quality in the health care they receive than in the automobiles they buy? This type of automated information system will greatly enhance and streamline the quality assurance process in the hospital and will generate data to allow providers to plan for the most efficient use of resources.

REFERENCES

Aydelotte, M. K., & Tener, M. E. (1960). *An investigation of the relation between nursing activity and patient welfare.* Iowa City: The University of Iowa.

Mowry, M. M., & Korpman, R. A. (1986). *Managing health care costs, quality and technology: Product line strategies for nursing.* Rockville, MD: Aspen.

O'Leary, D. (1987). The Joint Commission looks to the future. *Journal of the American Medical Association, 258,* 951-952.

Wyszewianski, L. (1988). Quality of care: Past achievements and future challenges. *Inquiry, 25,* 13-22.

CHAPTER 12

Health Care Technology and Quality of Care

Ada Jacox and Barbara Pillar

The relationship between technology used and quality of service delivered is increasingly important in the era of cost containment and competition. Current perspectives on technology assessment in health care focus attention on the relationship between technology assessment and quality assessment. Outcome measures to be considered in the evaluation of technology include safety and effectiveness, costs and benefits, and social impact. A discussion of technology assessment at the hospital level and within the nursing department allows for the identification of areas of concern for the nurse administrator. These include the need to determine the role of health care personnel and the impact of technology on nurses.

Health care technology is a major component of the delivery of health care services. It plays a prominent role in prevention, diagnosis, treatment, and rehabilitation. Although technology has contributed greatly and sometimes dramatically to the well-being of the nation, its use also has been accompanied by ethical questions and economic concerns (Ginsberg, 1990). In this chapter, we first discuss the relationship between health care technology and quality of care gener-

Johns Hopkins University, Baltimore, MD 21205; National Institutes of Health, 9000 Rockville Pike, Bethesda, MD 20892.

Series on Nursing Administration — Volume III, 1992

ally, with attention to the process of technology assessment. We then consider those aspects of technology and the quality of nursing care that have particular relevance to nurse administrators. A key issue in all phases of the technology life cycle involves quality of care and its role in technology development, implementation, and evaluation.

DEFINING TECHNOLOGY AND QUALITY

Technology, in the broadest sense, is the practical application of science. In health care, technology refers to the drugs, devices, and procedures used in the delivery of health care and to the organizational or administrative systems that support its use, encompassing such items as artificial kidneys, monitoring devices, computers, or cyclosporin (Office of Technology Assessment [OTA], 1982). It also can include technical procedures, information systems, or work patterns such as the carotid artery by-pass graft, the DRG classification system, and primary nursing.

It is important to note that technology is not limited to the "high tech" areas of a hospital such as intensive care units, magnetic resonance imaging units, or surgery suites. Technology is a component of the general medical-surgical units, administrative offices, and emergency rooms. It exists outside the hospital also—in outpatient clinics, nursing homes, physicians' offices, and the private home by means of home health care.

The life cycle of technology extends through development and testing, implementation in the health care system, widespread diffusion, or possibly, discontinuation. According to the National Center for Health Care Technology (NCHCT), an "emerging" technology is one expected to be in use within 5 years, a "new" technology has just received approval from the Federal Food and Drug Administration and is beginning to diffuse throughout the system, and an "established" technology is one that is in widespread use (NCHCT, 1980). Each stage brings new and varied issues for resource planning, continuing education for clinicians, and choices among competing technologies.

Quality in health care is more difficult to define and has been the subject of extensive research and speculation (Perry & Pillar, 1988). In the early work of Donabedian (1966), a proposal for a systematic approach to quality assessment focused on the structure of the system, on the process of delivering care, and on clinical and organizational outcomes. This conceptual framework still provides a useful and comprehensive approach to evaluating quality, although further work in this area has revealed specific additional elements that need to be assessed, including the following:

- Efficacy and effectiveness that reflect differences in the performance of a technology under ideal and normal conditions, respectively

- Appropriate use—the standard for clinical use of a technology that in some circumstances may raise ethical and legal considerations
- Caring—the element of human regard, compassion, and appreciation of individuality
- Efficiency—focusing on the best economic use of resources

Whatever framework or components are selected for evaluation, quality of care is defined as that attribute of care that signifies a grade of excellence. Donabedian (1980a) views quality as the extent to which care achieves the most favorable balance of risks and benefits; he defines cost, accessibility, continuity, and coordination as elements of care that influence quality. Emphasis is placed on the weighing of benefits against harm, efficiency, and economic costs.

The American Medical Association defines high-quality care as that "which consistently contributes to improvement or maintenance of the quality and/or duration of life" (Steffen, 1988). Quality of care is integrally related to favorable—that is, successful—patient outcomes. In nursing care the characteristics of quality often are expressed as "standards," which extends the definition of quality to include effectiveness (Van Maanen, 1984). Furthermore, the model for quality assurance developed by the American Nurses' Association is developed from a concept of quality that encompasses social, institutional, and individual values (Lang & Clinton, 1984).

From a different perspective, quality is not considered a property at all but is "the capacity to achieve goals" (Steffen, 1988). This approach is unique in its implication that preferences and values are intrinsically a part of an evaluation of quality. By including preferences and values, it admits the possibility of differences in goals between the patient and the health care professional, as well as acknowledging the existence of medical and nonmedical goals for both. Thus the quality of health care in any system would be affected if there were a discrepancy between the objectives of the parties involved.

A new federal agency established in 1989, the Agency for Health Care Policy and Research (AHCPR), has goals directly related to the provision of quality of care. These goals include (1) promoting improvements in clinical practice and patient outcomes through more appropriate and effective health care services, (2) promoting improvements in the financing, organization, and delivery of health care services, and (3) increasing access to quality care. The legislation established, within the agency, the Office of the Forum of Quality and Effectiveness in Health Care, which is responsible for facilitating the development, the review, and the updating of clinically relevant guidelines to assist health care practitioners in the prevention, diagnosis, treatment, and management of clinical conditions. The Office of the Forum "is responsible for developing a system of performance measures, standards of quality, and review criteria through which health care practitioners and others may review the provision of health care and assure its quality. Guidelines, standards, performance measures, and review criteria are to be based on the best available research and professional judgment regarding the effectiveness and appropriateness of health care services and procedures" (AHCPR, 1990).

This new federal agency clearly will have a major federal role in addressing issues of quality of care. Four of the 17 members of the advisory council to the agency are nurses, and three of the initial seven panels to develop clinical practice guidelines are chaired or cochaired by nurses.

Although there is no single, accepted definition of quality, it can be said that the attainment of quality of care is an objective, an ongoing, and a never-to-be-completed mission, much like the pursuit of clinical knowledge and skill. As advances occur in diagnostic and therapeutic health care and in methods of delivering care, more is learned about evaluating the implications of the results. In turn, additional problems, omissions, and errors are identified. The process of assessing quality also improves over time. Most recently, the introduction of continuous quality improvement has fostered an emphasis on patient needs and outcomes in order to increase the effectiveness of quality assurance programs (*Journal of Nursing Quality Assurance*, 1990).

The *pursuit* of quality is the focus of quality assurance efforts, and the *measurement* of quality is the objective of quality assessment. Quality assurance should "objectively and systematically monitor and evaluate the quality and appropriateness of patient care, pursue opportunities to improve patient care, and resolve identified problems" (Joint Commission, 1987). The quality assurance program of an institution generally serves as the primary initiator and coordinator of related activities such as quality assessment, utilization review, and peer review.

Other activities related to quality assurance, however, have not developed close links to the traditional quality-of-care framework. For example, risk assessment and management have been defined narrowly as the science for the identification, evaluation, and treatment of the risk of financial loss, focusing primarily on prevention of patient injuries (ECRI, 1987), and only recently have been linked to quality assessment activities (Youngberg, 1990). Even more significant has been the failure to recognize explicitly the critical importance of quality assessment and the evaluation of technologies through a process called *technology assessment.*

The ultimate purpose of evaluating health care technologies is to enhance quality of care, which is achieved through the development of standards and subsequent improved use of technologies. Because of this common goal, technology assessment is integrally related to quality assessment. Technology assessment is defined as a "form of research, analysis, and evaluation that attempts to examine the various impacts of a particular technology on the individual and society in terms of the technology's safety, efficacy, effectiveness, and cost effectiveness, and its social, economic, and ethical implications, and to identify those areas requiring further research, demonstrations, or evaluation" (NCHCT, 1981). From this research come the criteria and standards for the appropriate use of technology in the clinical setting. These criteria and standards form the basis for measurement in quality assessment. Thus there is a fundamental relationship, through a common purpose, between technology assessment, which sets standards, and quality assessment, which evaluates the extent to which the preset criteria and standards have been observed (Donabedian, 1987).

As previously noted, the quality assessment model views health care in terms of structure, process, and outcome. Technologies — whether drugs, devices, procedures, or organizational support systems — are the tools of health care and, as such, can be considered an essential part of the structure and process of the health care delivery system.

QUALITY ASSESSMENT AND TECHNOLOGY ASSESSMENT

A study by the Office of Technology Assessment (1988) on the quality of health care reported the following conclusion:

> Technology assessment should undergird assessment of the quality of a provider's practice. Using standards to evaluate the quality of care delivered to a patient requires that a quality assessor have criteria by which to judge how a particular condition is managed. The development of such criteria, in turn, should be based on knowledge about the efficacy and safety of new and existing technologies.

Technology assessment is a form of policy research that provides a mechanism for the health care professions to scrutinize technologies and to foster their appropriate use (Perry & Chu, 1986). The analysis of health effects resulting from the application of technology assists decision makers in establishing clinical or social policy. The assessment process is not intended to control the costs or diffusion of technologies. Rather technology assessment provides data and information for use by health care providers, decision makers, third-party payers, and others. Such information, particularly on the appropriate use of technology, should be integrated into quality assurance efforts.

Quality assessment and technology assessment share a concern with levels of performance of both the health care practitioner and the team or organization that provides the care. The two processes also seek to measure the impact of care delivered on the health of the individual and on the health of the community, focusing on two levels of quality. Both processes focus on assessing the immediate effects on the patient, as well as the long-range effects on the health care system.

There is increasing recognition that quality assessment and technology assessment are critically linked (Lohr & Rettig, 1988). In 1988 the Council of Health Care Technology of the Institute of Medicine sponsored a conference to consider the relationship between technology assessment and quality of care, observing that the fields have developed as separate endeavors, with different vocabularies, different methods, and under the leadership of different theoreticians and practitioners.

At the conference Robert Brook made the following observations (Brook, 1988):

- The quality and technology assessment fields perceive themselves to be different; they are, however, similar and integratively linked.
- Both quality and technology assessments require and depend on a broad definition of health.
- Both fields make evaluative judgments.
- For constructive action to occur, both fields must establish causal links between the process of care and patient outcomes.
- Measurement of cost is not sufficient to separate the fields.

Nurses generally have not been involved in the emerging field of technology assessment. This lack of involvement is reflected in the proceedings of the aforementioned conference, which are oriented primarily toward the relationship between health care technology and medical care and its impact on quality of patient care.

One of the presenters at the conference was interested in understanding the origin of the effort to relate technology assessment and quality of care. Gronvall (1988) noted that the connection was first documented in a paper by Florence Nightingale, published in 1859. The paper reflects Nightingale's concern with collecting accurate hospital statistics and with documenting the relationship between differences in patient characteristics, including the observation that "the elements which really give information . . . are those which show the proportion of sick restored to health, and the average time which has been required for this object. . . . the proportion of recoveries, the proportion of deaths, and the average time in hospital must all be taken in account . . . as well as the character of the cases and the proportion of different ages." Gronvall (1988) noted his fascination at hearing people call John Bunker "the father of us all," saying, "Now, I suppose, we also know who our mother is!"

TECHNOLOGY EVALUATION

For comprehensive evaluation of a technology, the following outcome measures are needed.

Safety and effectiveness. Safety and effectiveness are of primary concern because there are side effects to almost every drug and procedure and to some organizational support systems (IOM, 1985; OTA, 1978; OTA,

1982). Safety is a judgment of the acceptability of risk in a specified situation as calculated in a risk-to-benefit ratio, with risk being the number and severity of negative side effects or complications. In the estimation of safety, a low risk may be unacceptable if there is a small benefit, but a high risk may be acceptable if the benefit also is high.

Patient outcome is the endpoint in assessments of efficacy, which is the probability of benefit to individuals in a defined population under ideal conditions. A second measure is effectiveness, the probability of benefit of a technology under average conditions of use. Nursing treatment of decubitus ulcers, as administered under the controlled conditions of a research study to a selected sample, may not produce the same patient outcome in a general medical unit or in a nursing home. The most valid method of assessing safety and effectiveness is the randomized clinical trial, but other approaches, such as epidemiologic studies, technology case studies, and consensus development conferences, also are of value.

Costs and benefits. Methods that determine economic effects of health care technology are used to compare the positive and negative consequences of alternative ways to allocate resources. The primary techniques employed are cost-benefit analysis (CBA) and cost-effectiveness analysis (CEA). The difference between the two methods is that CBA measures all costs and benefits in monetary terms whereas CEA produces a measure of the benefits not in dollars but in some health-related effects such as added years of life. In other respects, the methods are similar (Phelps & Mushlin, 1991).

Economic analysis must take into account both the direct costs of health care, such as physician fees, nursing care, and supplies, and indirect costs such as the value of work time lost by the patient. In addition, cost analyses develop information on opportunity costs, production costs, research and development costs, overhead, and marginal valuation. Because of the complexities involved, the quality of the analysis depends on the assumptions made and the quality of the data. The calculation of costs and benefits or effectiveness associated with a technology is not always a component of the assessment of technologies. A review of CBA/CEA methods led the Office of Technology Assessment (1980) to conclude that an analysis of costs and benefits could be very helpful to decision makers. There are, however, too many limitations in both the CBA and CEA methods to justify their use as sole or prime determinants in decision making.

Social impact. The growth of health care technology has raised a number of social questions, as illustrated by the issues surrounding organ transplantation, equitable allocation of resources, surrogate motherhood, and prolongation of life in the seriously ill. The issues may be legal, ethical, or political and may involve the individual, family, health care system, or society as a whole. Legal questions may involve the negative consequences of medical and nursing care, such as iatrogenic injury, or the right to receive services paid for by insurers, such as renal dialysis. Ethical issues encompass protection of the very young and very old, equitable allocation of resources, and the application of benevolence and mercy.

As the technology in health care becomes more complex, it appears that the ethical issues become more complex. Nurses may become involved at all levels of decision making but often play a crucial role in the support of the patient and family caught up in a moral dilemma. In a recent discussion of terminating treatment in a neonatal intensive care unit, it was emphasized that parents need to understand that only extraordinary measures will be stopped but that nursing care and pain relief will be guaranteed (Raivio, 1991). Such reassurance must be conveyed by the nursing staff.

Use of Group Judgment

Technology assessment provides a research framework for organizing the various questions surrounding the study of technology. New or unique methods are not always required for such research inasmuch as numerous techniques from experimental, clinical, economic, legal, psychologic, and sociologic research are applicable to the study of health care technology. At the same time, new approaches such as meta-analysis, a method of aggregating data from multiple research studies, can contribute to technology assessment. Other approaches include studies of small area practice variations (Wennberg, 1984) and use of group judgment methods to determine appropriateness of procedures (Chassin et al., 1989).

An important method of group judgment is consensus development, a process whereby the biomedical research community, health care professionals, and others join to assess a technology to make certain it has been validated for safety and efficacy (Perry, 1987). It is aimed at a critical assessment of the current state of knowledge of what is known and what is not known, with the objective of affording the patient the optimal diagnostic approach and therapy available. Consensus development is directed particularly at emerging and new technologies that are controversial or about which there is confusion in the health care community. Examples of consensus conferences conducted at the National Institutes of Health (NIH, 1984-1991) include total hip replacement, ultrasound imaging in pregnancy, gastrointestinal surgery for severe obesity, and early stage breast cancer. Some conferences have focused on health problems such as geriatric assessment methods, diet and exercise in noninsulin-dependent diabetes, and osteoporosis.

Other group judgment techniques also have been used to advantage in assessing technology. Examples are the Delphi method, small working panels, and the "technology assessment forum" in which the product is a set of recommendations concerning the application of a technology based on a careful examination of the state-of-the-art. These approaches do not attempt to achieve consensus (Perry & Eliastam, 1981). A recent example is the small panel studies conducted by the Rand Corporation to determine the clinical indications for procedures such as coronary angiography, cholecystectomy, and colonoscopy (Park et al., 1986). Consensus development and other group judgment techniques are particularly applicable for quality assurance because they allow for the participation of diverse groups such as health care providers, consumers, ethicists, policy analysts, and other interested parties. Each has a useful contribution to make in providing a unique and important perspective to the process as it relates to fostering quality in health care.

Many of the characteristics of technology assessment make it a valuable research framework for nurses. The multidisciplinary approach ensures a comprehensive evaluation, and the use of methods such as randomized clinical trials and the use of consensus development ensure valid and useful outcomes. Furthermore, technology assessment, as a form of policy research, provides information on rational decision making. In health care the information obtained from evaluation may be used by lawmakers to formulate regulations and legislation for the health care industry, by health professionals in treating and caring for patients, by industry in developing products, and by consumers in making personal health decisions.

TECHNOLOGY ASSESSMENT AT THE HOSPITAL LEVEL

Understanding the similarities in quality assurance and technology assessment makes more clear the implications for the implementation of technology assessment activities at the hospital level and how such activities can be related to other activities. As noted earlier, one difference between the two fields is the emphasis placed in technology assessment on cost, an increasing concern in health care. Moxley (1988), president of a hospital chain, observed that expenditures for new and replacement technology will be reduced and that hospitals will be forced to become increasingly conservative purchasers. He reported that both the Hospital Corporation of America and American Medical International, Incorporated, reduced capital expenditures by at least 50% from 1985 to 1986, reflecting changes taking place throughout the hospital industry. Moxley summarized issues important to hospital administrators. He indicated that hospital managers want (1) more information on how new technology will affect existing technology and the management of disease, (2) information on what is the proper treatment site for new technology, (3) guidelines for dissemination of technology, including when it is appropriate for community hospitals—compared with tertiary care centers—to introduce new technology, (4) better estimates of turnover time based on true technology innovations, and (5) the Health Care Financing Administration payment approval process streamlined and based on a more realistic payment level for approved and new technology.

Acknowledgment that expenditures for technology must be markedly reduced illustrates the importance of the cost component in technology assessment and underscores why technology assessment activities will be increasingly addressed at all levels, including that of the hospital.

A number of issues related to technology use must be addressed by the hospital or health care agency, including nursing activities related to technology assessment. One is determining the quality of care to be given in the institution, including the kinds of technology used. These policy decisions are closely linked to policies of third-party payers. The extent to which third-party payers, both government and private, limit resources for patient care directly affects the amount available for specific technologies, as well as for new and replacement technologies generally.

A related issue is third-party payers' increasing willingness to pay only for care received by their clients rather than subsidizing the care of other patients. The restricted ability of hospital managers to cross-subsidize results in greater attention to the amount of unreimbursed care that an agency is willing or able to provide. Provision of high-technology care to those unable to pay will become an increasingly difficult policy decision for administrators and will make very clear the major policy issues concerned with technology. Who receives care? What level of care? Who pays? Decisions regarding technology increasingly will take place within the context of the clients served, the sources of payment, overall resources available to the hospital, and, when appropriate, amount of profit desired.

Nurses, who generally comprise the largest group of health care providers in the hospital, must be part of the overall institutional consideration of these and related issues. They also must be concerned with mechanisms within the nursing department to address relationships between technology and quality of nursing care.

TECHNOLOGY AND QUALITY OF NURSING CARE

It cannot be assumed that more technology (in the narrow sense of equipment) means improved patient care. Technology in this sense is only one factor that influences patient care and may not even be the most important one, as illustrated in some important research (Knaus, Draper, Wagner, & Zimmerman, 1986).

In a study of nine ICUs in 13 hospitals, researchers developed a severity-of-disease classification system for critically ill adult patients to predict expected mortality. Using the APACHE II classification system to estimate expected mortality rates, they compared predicted with actual mortality rates and found that in the best functioning ICUs 41% fewer deaths than predicted occurred, whereas in the most poorly functioning units 58% more deaths occurred than predicted. They found no differences across units in the technology available, the amount of treatment received, or whether the ICU was in a teaching hospital: "Instead, hospital performances appeared to be related to the quality of the care delivering system as it pertained to the coordination and communication among and between nurses and physicians" (Draper, 1987, p. 7). In the best functioning units, nurses and physicians showed mutual respect and consulted each other in the care of patients. In the poorest functioning units, there were problems in communication between nurses and physicians, with the worst hospitals characterized by an atmosphere of mistrust, physicians who did not respect the nurses enough to communicate routinely with them during patient rounds, and nurses who were concerned about contacting physicians to clarify their orders because of fear of annoying or angering the physician. The study does not suggest that technology (hardware) is unimportant, because all ICUs had high levels of technology. It made clear, however, that organizational and social support aspects of technology can have a dramatic impact on quality of care.

On the basis of the broad definition of technology presented in this chapter, many of the usual concerns of nursing service administrators are inherent in dealing with technology and its relationship to quality of patient care. Two major interrelated concerns are determining the roles of various health care personnel so that cost-effective, quality care can be provided and considering the effects of high technology and inadequate staffing on patients and their families. An additional consideration is the impact of technology on nurses.

Roles of Health Care Personnel

With introduction of new technologies often comes introduction of new technicians to monitor the technology or to provide technology-related care. The Institute of Medicine (1989) released a report of "allied health" occupations, which listed nearly 150 different occupations. In the face of such proliferation of types of workers, long-standing issues related to who should provide what kinds of care to patients at the bedside and how the caregivers should be supervised and coordinated become paramount concerns. The problem is how to analyze health care delivery so that personnel with the requisite knowledge and skills deliver care to patients in the most efficient and least costly way. An attendant need is to strike a balance between workers with skills in fairly narrow areas and nurses who traditionally give more comprehensive patient care.

Recent attempts to reduce costs in hospitals have produced a number of ways of dealing with the multiple types of health care workers. Some hospitals, in moving to all-RN nursing staffs and reduction of support staff, have produced a situation in which RNs are expected to carry out nursing activities, as well as many housekeeping, clerical, and errand-type activities. This practice has resulted in underutilization of nurses' expertise and in dissatisfaction among nurses. Wan and Shukla (1987) reported no relationship between nursing staff skill mix (RN hours and LPN hours per patient day) or mode of patient care delivery (primary nursing vs. others) on adverse incident rates for patients (e.g., medication and IV line errors, patient falls and injuries). They explained the absence of relationship between nursing model and adverse incidents by noting that "primary nursing is effective only when support systems are efficient; when hospitals with inefficient support systems adopt a primary nursing model, they utilize registered nurses' skills poorly . . . " (Wan & Shukla, 1987, p. 64).

In other hospitals, a more thoughtful approach has been taken to reallocating responsibilities, such as one hospital's report on the integration of respiratory therapy into nursing (Watson & Strasen, 1987). After an analysis of the activities performed by respiratory therapists and nursing staff members, areas of duplication that were identified included (1) assessing and documenting patient conditions and responses, (2) ordering and distributing respiratory therapy supplies, and (3) distributing and billing for medications. The latter two functions were reassigned to central supply and pharmacy departments. Patient care activities were reassigned to the nursing staff, resulting in a decrease of 10 respiratory therapists and $270,000 of annual salary expense. The rationale for such reassignment of activities was that a professional, in this case the nurse, with a broader scope of activity could efficiently include aspects of practice such as respiratory therapy, thus increasing the productivity of nurses: "During respiratory therapy down time, nurses can perform several other tasks while respiratory therapists are limited in their scope of practice. Any ancillary department that provides service throughout a hospital spends a significant amount of time traveling to and from the patients. This reduces the time spent providing actual hands-on care to patients. However, when the primary licensed nurse caring for the patient provides the service, nonproductive time is essentially eliminated . . ." (Watson & Strasen, 1987). This kind of careful planning across departments, as well as within nursing, needs to occur to provide quality patient care within the context of increased technology and cost constraints.

Effects of High Technology on Patients and Need for Support

Concern with providing supportive patient care is critical in considering the relationship between technology and quality of nursing care. Many of the numerous personnel at the patient's bedside are concerned with monitoring parts of the machinery or with providing limited services, making it even more important that nurses attend to a broad range of patient needs, including provision of comfort and support to the patient and family. The anxiety evoked for hospitalized patients and their families is exacerbated by the complex monitoring and treatment devices that flash, buzz, or otherwise make their presence known. Studies have documented the high noise levels in critical care units, for example, and their negative effects on patients (Baker, 1984; Hansell, 1984). The importance of giving patients and their families explanations regarding the technology and providing comfort and emotional support cannot be overstated.

The relationship between numbers and types of nursing personnel, what they do with patients, and the effect on patient outcomes is complex and has received little study. That such studies are needed is increasingly apparent.

An article in the *Washington Post* ("Questions raised," 1989), for example, reported on a for-profit community hospital being scrutinized by state and federal health officials who were threatening to revoke the hospital's Medicare privilege. Incidents cited in the articles included one of an RN who administered an intravenous injection of potassium instead of furosemide, which resulted in the patient's death. According to the nurse involved, the two drugs were stored side by side on a shelf, and "a lot of nights I was the only RN . . . there. . . . You were overloaded when you were working there. . . . The hospital was 'very dangerous' and 'not what it should be' " ("Questions raised," p. 27).

As nurse executives are able to demonstrate that inadequate numbers and types of nursing personnel produce an inadequate quality of care, it should increase the ability to negotiate more favorably on behalf of the nursing department.

Impact of High Technology on Nursing Personnel

Except for concerns with such things as work-related injuries or exposure to infectious diseases, occupational health hazards in hospitals and other settings in which nurses work have received little attention. In recent years the Occupational Safety and Health Association (OSHA) has begun to focus on such hazards for nursing, including stress in the work environment (Williamson et al., 1988). Stress is related to caring for sick and dying people, heavy workloads, noise, and other factors, as well as interacting in a highly charged and frequently volatile work environment. Contemporary hospitals are increasingly characterized by high technology in intensive care and telemetry units, as well as in those units not usually thought of as "high tech." Because of the necessity to know how to respond both to the patient and to the technology surrounding the patient during the crises that are common in hospitals, the stress level for nurses is high and the consequences of making mistakes are serious.

A study of noise-induced stress in critical care nurses identified that the top three disturbing noises for nurses were beeping monitors, equipment alarms, and ringing telephones (Topf & Dillon, 1988). Less distressful noises included the intercom and call lights, hematocrit spinner, background conversations during report, falling objects such as pans and charts, and ventilators. The authors interpreted the findings to mean that "nurses were bothered most by equipment noises signaling that action should be taken." They noted that critical care nurses are exposed to unpredictable and inescapable noises from a variety of equipment sources on a long-term basis and that noise-induced stress is related to burnout.

Compounding the technologic complexity is the current concern with acquired immunodeficiency syndrome (AIDS) and other infectious diseases to which nurses frequently are exposed. This necessitates additional precautions for protection of personnel, but the technology for self-protection remains controversial. All these factors take their toll on nursing personnel.

Identification of stressors and their effects on nurses is important in understanding how the work environment may be modified to reduce the cumulative stress. Keane and Adler (1985), for example, found that the quality of hardiness reduced the probability of burnout or feelings of powerlessness. Their study, as well as others, described the burnout that results from feelings of powerlessness in not being able to manage job responsibilities because of factors beyond the control of nurses. Although the ability to deal with stress varies considerably among nurses, nurse executives can acknowledge and help their staff members deal with high stress levels by taking actions such as the following: (1) developing mechanisms to increase nurses' involvement in decisions regarding patient care and working conditions, (2) structuring nursing personnel's assignments so that periods of work in high stress areas are relieved by spending time in some units in which the pace is less hectic and demanding, (3) modifying the physical environment to reduce noise levels, and (4) finding effective ways to understand and interpret the effects of inadequate staffing on nurses and on patient outcomes.

TECHNOLOGY ASSESSMENT WITHIN THE NURSING DEPARTMENT

It is important that technology assessment activities be formally located in the organization and that they be related to other similar activities. Increasingly, nurse executives recognize the need for organizational units with staff members who can perform needed research-related activities, including research, quality assurance, program evaluation, monitoring compliance with clinical practice guidelines and standards, and technology assessment. It is becoming a more common practice to assign such units to nurse administrators with backgrounds in research.

Although responsibility for conducting technology assessment activities may be placed in an existing research and development department, there also is a need to involve other professionals and administrators with varying types of knowledge. This includes persons knowledgeable about the financial operations of the hospital and how to address the cost issues in technology assessment, which requires expertise about hospital cost-accounting measures, as well as understanding of cost-effectiveness analysis. If nursing personnel do not have such knowledge, consultants need to be included in planning technology assessment activities. Consultation with others also is needed when decisions are made regarding who will carry out the activities related to technology. In the earlier example of the integration of respiratory therapy skills as part of nursing care, nurses, inhalation therapists, hospital administrators, pharmacists, and central supply, representatives were involved in deciding how activities would be relocated and what might be the organizational consequences of such reassignment. An article (Jacox, Pillar, & Redman, 1990) on classification of nursing technology illustrates the broad overlap across health care occupations in use of technology and underscores the need for an interdisciplinary approach in its assessment. Another kind of knowledge required in technology assessment, often on an ad hoc basis, is that of the clinicians who are or who will become expert in the use of the technology being evaluated. We all have experienced or heard accounts of the negative organizational consequences of computer systems, monitoring equipment, or other sophisticated technology being introduced without input from nurses or others who are to be responsible for using the technology and for caring for the patient receiving it. The need in technology assessment for persons with various kinds of knowledge is apparent in the kinds of issues addressed.

Assuming the availability of personnel with requisite types of knowledge, one of the first functions in establishing a technology assessment program is to establish criteria for priorities in evaluating technology. At the national level the Institute of Medicine (Lara & Goodman, 1990) identified the following primary criteria for selecting clinical conditions or technologies for assessment: potential to improve individual patient outcome, potential to affect a large patient population, potential to reduce unit or aggregate cost, and potential to reduce unexplained variations in medical practice. Nursing needs to undertake the same kind of activity in deciding which aspects of technology will be assessed and when. Criteria to be considered focus on the following questions. (1) How common is the technology? (2) How costly is it? (3) What is the error rate associated with its use? (4) What areas represent conflicting opinions with regard to how care ought to be delivered? (5) What is the potential impact on patients? (6) How nursing resource–intense is it?

These and similar criteria should provide some guidance to assessment staff members in their evaluation of both new and existing technologies. Further, evaluation of existing technology requires attention to questions such as the following. Which patients should receive a particular form of hardware, for example, specialty beds, IV monitors, infusion pumps for patient-controlled analgesia, and electronic monitoring of vital signs? Should all patients on a nursing unit have them, or should their use be limited to patients with specific needs or those who are at risk for particular problems? Considering the organizational aspects of technology, relevant concerns relate to the choice of nursing care delivery modes. Under what circumstances, for example, is primary nursing the mode of choice, and when might a case management system or a team approach be more efficient and effective? Another factor to consider is identification of technologies that have a potentially negative effect on nursing personnel. The current concern with AIDS, for example, makes clear the need to understand safety precautions in handling infectious materials. The negative effects on nurses of being required to perform many nonnursing housekeeping and clerical tasks under various modes of nursing service delivery have been previously noted. The impact of technologies on those delivering them is a part of technology assessment that often is overlooked.

Through some sort of consensus process, decisions should be reached regarding which technologies and aspects of technology assessment need to be addressed further. The next step is to review existing evidence with regard to the safety, efficacy, efficiency, and cost of the technology, including evidence in the literature, as well as that available through hospital sources knowledgeable about the technology. Data can be collected from nurses and others using the technology, as well as from patients who are receiving it. Depending on the technology to be assessed, appropriate methods of conducting the assessment are selected from those identified earlier in this chapter. Finally, once the technology has been implemented, there is need to monitor or audit its use to ensure that the technology is being implemented correctly and that it is having the desired effect on patient care and costs.

CONCLUSION

This chapter has focused on health care technology and quality of care, first from a broad perspective and then specifically related to nursing. It can be anticipated that concern with the relationship between technology and quality of care will increase in significance for nurse administrators operating in a cost conscious environment. It is imperative that nursing departments have within them personnel with the requisite knowledge and skills to document and interpret the relationship between health care technology and quality of nursing care.

REFERENCES

Agency for Health Care Policy and Research. (1990). *AHCPR program note: Clinical guideline development.* Rockville, MD: Author.

Baker, C. (1984). Sensory overload and noise in the ICU: Sources of environmental stress. *Critical Care Quarterly, 6,* 66-80.

Brook, R. H. (1988). Quality assessment and technology assessment: Critical linkages. In K. N. Lohr & R. A. Rettig (Eds.), *Quality of care and technology assessment* (pp. 26-27). Washington, DC: Institute of Medicine–National Academy Press.

Chassin, M. R., Kosecoff, J., Park, R. E., Winslow, C. M., Kahn, K. L., Merrick, N. J., Fink, A., Keesey, J., Solomon, D. H., & Brook, R. H. (1989). *The appropriateness of selected medical and surgical procedures: Relationship to geographical variations.* Ann Arbor, MI: Association for Health Services Research and Health Administration Press.

Donabedian, A. (1966). Evaluating the quality of medical care. *Milbank Memorial Fund Quarterly, 44,* 166-206.

Donabedian, A. (1980). *The definition of quality and approaches to its assessment.* Ann Arbor, MI: Health Administration Press.

Donabedian, A. (1987, May 21-22). *The assessments of technology and quality: A comparative study of certainties and ambiguities.* Paper presented at the Third Annual Meeting of the International Society for Technology Assessment in Health Care. Rotterdam, The Netherlands.

Draper, E. A. (1987). Effects of nurse/physician collaboration and nursing standards on ICU patients' outcomes. *Current Concepts in Nursing, 1*(4), 2-9.

ECRI. (1987). Quality of care and technology. *Health Technology, 1*(5), 191-198.

Ginsberg, E. (1990). High-tech medicine and risking health care costs. *Journal of the American Medical Association, 263*(13), 190-195.

Gronvall, J. A. (1988). The view of a government medical care provider, quality assurer, and technology assessor. In K. N. Lohr & R. A. Rettig (Eds.), *Quality of care and technology assessment* (pp. 126-133). Washington, DC: Institute of Medicine: National Academy Press.

Hansell, H. (1984). The behavioral effects of noise on man: The patient with "intensive care unit psychosis." *Heart and Lung, 13,* 59-65.

Institute of Medicine. (1985). The scope of U.S. medical technology assessment. In *Assessing medical technologies.* Washington, DC: National Academy Press.

Institute of Medicine. (1989). *Allied health services: Avoiding crises.* Washington, DC: National Academy Press.

Jacox, A., Pillar, B., & Redman, B. K. (1990). A classification of nursing technology. *Nursing Outlook, 28*(2), 81-85.

Joint Commission on Accreditation of Hospitals. (1987). *Accreditation manual for hospitals.* Chicago: Author.

Journal of Nursing Quality Assurance. (1990). Quality, appropriateness, and continuous improvement. *5*(1), vi, 1-90.

Keane, D., & Adler, D. (1985). Stress in ICU and non-ICU nurses. *Nursing Research, 34,* 231-236.

Knaus, W., Draper, E., Wagner, D., & Zimmerman, Y. (1986). An evaluation of outcome from intensive care in major medical centers. *Annals of Internal Medicine, 104,* 410-418.

Lang, N., & Clinton, J. F. (1984). Quality assurance: the idea and development of in the United States. In L. D. Willis & M. E. Linwood (Eds.), *Recent advances in nursing: Vol. 10. Measuring the quality of care.* New York: Churchill-Livingstone.

Lara, M. L., & Goodman, C. (Eds.) (1990). *National priorities for the assessment of clinical conditions and medical technologies: Priority setting group* (Council on Health Care Technology). Washington, DC: Institute of Medicine: National Academy Press.

Lohr, K. N., & Rettig, R. A. (Eds.) (1988). *Quality of care and technology assessment.* Washington, DC: Institute of Medicine: National Academy Press.

Moxley, J. H. III. (1988). Technology assessment: view of a multihospital system. In K. N. Lohr & R. A. Rettig (Eds.), *Quality of care and technology assessment* (pp. 89-97). Washington, DC: Institute of Medicine: National Academy Press.

National Center for Health Care Technology. (1980). *Guidance document for preparation of the emerging technology list: Internal memorandum*. Washington, DC: Author.

National Center for Health Care Technology. (1981). *Process for assessing technologies*. Washington, DC: Author.

National Institutes of Health. (1984-1991). *Consensus Development Conferences summary statements*. Washington, DC: Author.

Nightingale, F. (1982). Notes on hospitals: Being two papers read before the National Association for the Promotion of Social Science at Liverpool, in October, 1858. Birmingham, AL: The Classics of Medicine Library. (Facsimile reproduction of the work originally published in 1859.)

Office of Technology Assessment. (1978). *Assessing the safety and efficacy of medical technology* (Publication No. OTA-H-75). Washington, DC: U.S. Government Printing Office.

Office of Technology Assessment. (1980). *The implications of cost-effectiveness analysis of medical technology*. (Publication No. OTA-H-126). Washington, DC: U.S. Government Printing Office.

Office of Technology Assessment. (1982). *Strategies for medical technology assessment* (Publication No. OTA-H-181). Washington, DC: U.S. Government Printing Office.

Office of Technology Assessment. (1988). *The quality of medical care: Information for consumers*. (Publication No. OTA-H-387). Washington, DC: U.S. Government Printing Office.

Park, R. E., Fink, A., Brook, R., Chassin, M., Lahn, K., Merrick, N., Kosecoff, J., & Solomon, D. (1986). Physician ratings of appropriate indications for six medical and surgical procedures. *American Journal of Public Health, 76*, 766-772.

Perry S. (1987). The NIH consensus development program: A decade later. *New England Journal of Medicine, 317*, 485-488.

Perry, S., & Chu, F. (1986). The interrelationship between technology assessment, quality of care, and quality assurance. *Proceedings of an international symposium on quality assurance in health care*. Paris.

Perry, S., & Eliastam, M. (1981). The national center for health care technology. *Journal of the American Medical Association, 245*, 2510-2511.

Perry, S., & Pillar, B. (1988). *Technology assessment in the pursuit of quality of care*. Paper prepared for the Association of Academic Health Centers. Washington, DC.

Phelps, C. E., & Mushlin, A. I. (1991). On the (near) equivalence of cost-effectiveness and cost-benefit analyses. *International Journal of Technology Assessment in Health Care, 7*(1), 12-21.

Questions raised about quality of care at P. G. Hospital. (1989, February 5). *Washington Post*, pp. 26-28.

Raivio, K. O. (1991). Ethical problems in neonatal intensive care. *International Journal of Technology Assessment in Health Care, 7*(Suppl. 1), 136-138.

Steffen, G. (1988). Quality medical care: A definition. *Journal of the American Medical Association, 260*, 56-61.

Topf, M., & Dillon, E. (1988). Noise-induced stress as a predictor of burnout in critical care nurses. *Heart and Lung, 17*, 567-574.

Van Maanen, H. M. (1984). Evaluation of nursing care: A multinational perspective. In L. D. Willis & M. E. Linwood (Eds.). *Recent advances in nursing: Vol. 10. Measuring the quality of care*. New York: Churchill-Livingstone.

Wan, T. H., & Shukla, R. K. (1987). Contextual and organizational correlates of the quality of hospital nursing care. *Quality Review Bulletin, 13*, 61-64.

Watson, D., & Strasen, L. (1987). The integration of respiratory therapy into nursing: Reorganization for improved productivity. *Hospital and Health Services Administration, 32,* 369-377.

Wennberg, J. E. (1984). Dealing with medical practice variations: A proposal for action. *Health Affairs, 3*(2), 6-32.

Williamson, K. M., Turner, J. G., Brown, K. C., Newman, K. D., Sirles, A. T., & Selleck, C. S. (1988). Occupational health hazards for nurses. II. *Image, 20*(3), 162-168.

Youngberg, B. J. (1990). *Essentials of hospital risk management.* Rockville, MD: Aspen Publishers.

CHAPTER 13

Nursing Research
and Quality Care

Cheryl B. Stetler

Research and quality assurance that relies on evaluation have a common base in the application of problem-solving approaches. Research activities, including research utilization, can contribute to quality assurance activities by generating knowledge, methods, and instruments, as well as by increasing the analytic skills of staff members. Quality assurance also can contribute to the research process through problem identification. A number of methods have been proposed for integrating research, clinical practice, and evaluation. The challenge for nursing service administration is to provide mechanisms whereby the integration of research and the assurance of quality can take place.

Today's nursing service administrator is expected to oversee the delivery of "safe, efficient, [and] cost-effective care" to a defined population of recipients (ANA Task Force, 1988, p. 1). Quality is of course an inherent component of this expectation, and quality assurance programs are a fixture in organized nursing services. A second, increasingly recognized, component of the safe, efficient, and cost-effective delivery of nursing care is research, also now included in standards for organized nursing services (ANA Task Force, 1988). Research, however, is

Hartford Hospital, 80 Seymour Street, Hartford, CT 06115.

Series on Nursing Administration – Volume III, 1992

not yet widely incorporated as an activity that can affect quality on either a long-term or a daily operational level.

The challenge for nursing service administrators is to provide mechanisms for the systematic, ongoing, and realistic integration of research and assurance of quality. In order for this to happen, these individual concepts and related activities must be well understood (Peters & Pearlson, 1989; Stetler, 1984). In turn, explicit decisions must be made relative to expectations for the performance of personnel and investment of needed resources. Of central importance in this integrative process is the perception of research beyond its traditional image, that is, as the *conduct* of formalized studies.

A broader concept is required, which incorporates research as an integral component of critical thinking; as a process that can influence how well managers, clinicians, and educators solve problems on a day-to-day basis; as an entity that provides strategies for improvement of routine decision making; and, overall, as a means to search continually for quality improvements and excellence. Explicit strategies for *utilization* of research must therefore also be developed and implemented, or the potential for research to enhance quality will not be realized.

This chapter first explores the meaning of the term *research* and its relationship to quality and quality improvement. Next, problems of ambiguity created by varying usage of terms are described. Finally, a model is presented that integrates research and research utilization with the concept of quality, and related organizational implications are considered.

DEFINITIONS AND DISTINCTIONS

Over the past several years, nurses in various service settings have become increasingly interested in research. The predominant focus of this interest has been conducting research, particularly in relation to clinical practice (Hoare & Earenfight, 1986; Marchette, 1985; Reeves, Underly, & Beckwith, 1982; Rizzuto & Mitchell, 1988; Scogna, 1981). One rationale cited for the development of these clinically based research programs is their contribution to the scientific base of nursing practice. Implicitly, of course, the acquisition of scientific knowledge that contributes to the base for practice should over time enhance quality through the accumulation of replicated findings. Yet the fact that research has such a long-term perspective, whereas nurses in the service setting often wish to solve immediate problems, leads to inevitable questions regarding the relationship between the conduct of clinical research and the formal assurance of quality (Beyers, 1988; Kerfoot & Watson, 1985; Larson, 1983; Lieske, 1985; Peters & Pearlson, 1989).

Quality and research may appear to deal with distinctly different processes.

- Research can be defined as the scientific method of problem solving utilized for the purposes of describing, predicting, and controlling phenomena in our environment. It is concerned with the ultimate purpose of theory building (Holzemer, 1980; Isaac & Michael, 1982; Kerlinger, 1964; Polit & Hungler, 1991).
- Quality, according to a dictionary definition, means degree of excellence. It can be described in terms of effectiveness and efficiency (Luker, 1981), benefits and harm (Wyszewianski, 1988), or appropriateness of care (Berwick, 1989; Leape, 1990). A related definition is that "quality looks at how well policies, procedures, practices, and standards are carried out on behalf of an individual patient and groups of patients" (Patterson, 1988, p. 631). Within the service setting the concern is whether "quality"—that is, effectiveness, efficiency, and appropriateness—exists or to what degree there is inefficiency, poor execution, lack of effectiveness, or inappropriate care. The focus has thus been quality assurance, or most simply put, the assurance of the quality or excellence of care. Lieske (1985) further clarified quality assurance in nursing as "the process of evaluation applied to the health care system, and more specially to the provision of health care services by the professional nurse" (p. 194).

In the past few years, emphasis in this area has begun to move from the *assurance* of quality to continuous quality *improvement* or *management* (Nadzam, 1991; Sahney, Durkewych, & Schramm, 1989; Staff, 1990; also see Chapter 7 in this volume). Nonetheless, the fundamental focus for "quality" remains the same: the pursuit of excellence. (For purposes of the remainder of this chapter, the term "quality assurance" frequently will be used inasmuch as recent references still incorporate this terminology.)

In summary, the purpose of nursing research is generalizable knowledge, or theory building, whereas the focus of quality assurance, a form of evaluation, can be defined as "product delivery or mission accomplishment" in a specific setting (Isaac & Michael, 1982, p. 2). In the same vein, Wyszewianski (1988) points out that quality assurance activities are undertaken for the purpose of determining whether the right thing was done and done "right," whereas research (or studies of efficacy) determines what the right thing is!

Despite this identified distinction, difficulty arises when the assurance of quality or a program of improvement must be made operational in terms of various strategies of evaluation, a process that can be easily confused with research, particularly when its most formal state is known as evaluation research. (Woody [1980] believes the term *evaluation research* is in essence a contradiction in terms.) Further confusion can arise when the phrase *quality assurance study* is used. Kerfoot and Watson (1985), for example, attempted to clearly differentiate research and quality assurance "studies" through a set of criteria; for example, quality assurance studies were said to introduce interventions commonly accepted in practice whereas research focused on new nursing practices. Later in their article, however, the authors state that "the investigation of quality assurance problems must be viewed as quality assurance research" (p. 544).

A final methodology used for quality management (whose nomenclature is potentially confusing) is action research (Hunt, 1987). Webb (1989) describes action research as a process whereby nurses can "analyze problems, devise programmes of action designed to solve problems or improve standards, [and] carry out and evaluate these plans . . ." (p. 404). Lewin's conceptual basis for this activity involves a recurring cycle of "fact-finding, action and evaluation" (Webb, 1989, p. 405).

In reality, each—research, quality assurance, and evaluation—uses some type of problem-solving process. On the one hand, it can be argued that research is more formal and precise and that evaluation, unlike research, must focus on issues of worth, goal setting, and decision making. On the other hand, proponents of evaluative research or quality assurance studies cite methodologies reminiscent of those described in research texts and indeed may call for a similar level of precision (Holzemer, 1980; Kerfoot & Watson, 1985; Watson, Bulecheck, & McCloskey, 1987; Weiss, 1972). Because distinctions thereby become blurred, some authors have suggested that a continuum be visualized, with research on one end and evaluation on the other (Bloch, 1980; Luker, 1981). By means of this concept, one end of the continuum could be defined as highly controlled experimental research, with its formality and precision; at the other end could be day-to-day evaluation—one component of quality assurance—with its informality and, indeed, potential lack of precision. In the middle would be activities of a varying degree of rigor. Such an approach is conceptually appealing, but alone it does not provide a clear framework for explicating the relationship of research and quality or quality assurance improvement.

A MODEL FOR INTEGRATION

One term that does not frequently appear in the literature on quality is research utilization (RU). As already indicated, articles have appeared that attempt to differentiate research and quality assurance; few, however, explicitly focus on how *utilization* of the products and processes of research, rather than its conduct, can be put to work to enhance quality as an ongoing process. An exception is the quality assurance model using research (QAMUR) developed by Watson and associates (1987). This model incorporates both the conduct and utilization of research as critical components of a quality assurance program. Its focus, however, is on formal quality assurance studies that "should be done under the same stringent standards as nursing research" (p. 26). For the utilization component, the authors follow the organizationally oriented Conduct and Utilization of Research in Nursing (CURN) model (Horsley, Crane, & Bingle, 1978). This highly structured approach includes conduct of formal clinical trials. Although the QAMUR model is valuable, its focus is not broad enough to allow full realization of the potential for integration.

Table 13-1 presents an alternative model for the integration of research in the clinical setting. It provides a means to discuss the contribution that both research *and* its use can make to quality and the conduct of quality improvement activities.

Research

As already discussed, research is "directed toward the production of knowledge that is generalizable beyond the population directly studied" (Haller et al., 1979, p. 46). What that knowledge can provide is a scientific basis for the designation of quality. In fact, quality assurance activities "to be truly meaningful, require that it be known, a priori, what intervention is efficacious . . ." (Wyszewianski, 1988, p. 17). Nursing of course does not yet have the type of knowledge base that can provide the "right thing" to do in the multitude of situations that nurses encounter.

In 1980 Bloch called for "extensive testing of process-outcome relationships in current nursing practice, and development of methods for and testing of structure-process-outcome relationships" (p. 70). Such research continues to be a high-priority need. It is therefore critical that *conduct* of research be supported within the clinical setting so that the theoretic basis for provision of quality care can be continuously enhanced. Perhaps the lack of an in-depth knowledge base regarding nursing—from validation of nursing diagnoses to identification of effective interventions—has contributed to the confusion between quality assurance "studies" and research. Given the need for information on both efficacy and effectiveness, some individuals unwittingly end up by trying, unsuccessfully, to answer both simultaneously.

Another critical contribution that research can make to the definition and assessment of quality is development of related measuring methods and instruments (Bloch, 1980). As is clear from the remainder of this volume, quality is not a purely objective, scientifically based term and involves, to some extent, values, assumptions, choice, and judgment (Holzemer, 1980; Isaac & Michael, 1982; Staff, 1990). The existence of valid and reliable instruments, based on a clear conceptual framework, can facilitate the identification of assumptions and values. Also, development and testing of such instruments are extremely complex, time-consuming, and costly activities, which, however, researchers have the knowledge and skills to undertake.

TABLE 13-1   Research in the Service Setting

Research Utilization

Directed toward transferring specific research-based knowledge into actual
  practice (Haller et al., 1979)
Problem- and institution-focused

Types
1. Use of the research process
2. Use of research products

Focus

Process	Product
Routine data collection methods	Policy, procedure standards, and
Routine data collection tools	teaching tool development
Product evaluations	Routine problem solving, provi-
Introduction of innovations	sion of care or management
Program/project evaluations	Program development
	Instruments/tools for information
	gathering
	Technology decisions

Format
Variable, based on problem/need, ranging from informal to formal

Criteria of Acceptability

Process	Product
Objectivity, accuracy, clarity, and	Applicability criteria (see Stetler
credibility	and Marram, 1976; Horsley
Organizational relevance, priority,	et al., 1983)
and timeliness	Managerial/peer/relevant, commit-
Cost effectiveness	tee approval
Managerial/relevant, committee ap-	Fit/purpose of tool; reliability/
proval, and choice making	validity

Expectations
Ongoing, continuous improvement in practitioner and organizational
  functioning/goal achievement
Internal dissemination of results as required

Utilization

In contrast to research, utilization is "directed toward transferring
specific research-based knowledge into actual practice" (Haller et al.,
1979, p. 46). This can occur in one of two ways: (1) through utilization of
the end products of the conduct of research and (2) through utilization
of the concepts or methods of the research process (Stetler, 1985).

Utilization of research products. Three types of research products can
directly affect quality within the clinical setting: findings, measuring in-

---

Research

Directed toward the production of knowledge that is generalizable beyond the
   population directly studied (Haller et al., 1979)
Knowledge- and theory-focused

1. Nonexperimental   i. Replication
2. Quasiexperimental   ii. Original
3. Experimental

Research question/s
Research hypotheses

Complete scientific research proposal and report

Research committee review
   Scientific merit, e.g., control
   Administrative feasibility
Human subject protection
   Informed consent
   Subject protection and confidentiality

Addition to nursing's body of knowledge/theory base
Widespread dissemination of results
Scientific recognition/credibility

---

struments, and technologies. Results or findings of research can be used
both formally and informally to enhance the quality of care delivered;
whether the concern is structure, process, or outcome. In formal terms,
all clinical settings are expected to have policies, procedures, and standards of care in place (Patterson, 1988). Many patient teaching tools,
discharge plans, practice guidelines, protocols, and other documents that
support practice also are developed in many clinical settings, in which
models of care delivery, patient education programs, orientation pro-

grams for new graduates, and a variety of other programs for patient care and management of the nursing staff care are created.

A question, however, can be raised regarding how consistently, consciously, and knowledgeably groups assigned to develop such documents and programs utilize research-based literature. This question also applies to the less formal but quality-relevant situations that occur as clinical nurse specialists, staff educators, or nurse managers make decisions, provide consultations, model care, manage practice, educate staff members, or attempt to persuade others of the value of various programs or choices.

Studies within nursing over the past 10 years indicate some progress in the general effect of research on practice (see the results of Hefferin, Horsley, & Ventura, 1982; Kirchhoff, 1982; and Stokes, 1981, vs. those of Brett, 1987; Coyle & Sokop, 1990; and Stetler & DiMaggio, 1991). More progress, however, certainly is required as indicated both by the aforementioned findings and by the number of pragmatic articles continuing to encourage systematic utilization of research in practice (Briones & Bruya, 1990; Gaits et al., 1989; Lindquist, Brauer, Lekander, & Foster, 1990). This usage is particularly important as an expanding base of research is becoming available, and publications devoted specifically to the dissemination and discussion of research relevant to nurse clinicians, educators, and managers are continuing to appear.*

Research findings can provide a rationale and framework for the development of formal, "effective" documents and programs (see Goode, Lovett, Hayes, & Butcher, 1987). They also can influence an individual's quality of daily practice and management through provision of a scientific knowledge base that effects some of the following results (Stetler, 1985; Stetler & DiMaggio, in press; Stetler & Marram, 1976; Van Servellan & Stetler, 1986; Wiese, 1989):

- Enhances understanding or awareness of issues or problems
- Enhances identification of potential patient interventions or managerial strategies
- Facilitates evaluation of ongoing care and patient progress
- Supports actions or proposals about which others must be persuaded of the value or validity

As Cronenwett (1987) further suggests, through exposure to research findings, nurses can "improve the quality of assessment of a problem, analyze an intervention from a new perspective, or gain an increased awareness of the link between nursing care and patient outcome" (p. 9).

Utilization of research findings requires specific knowledge and skills,

---

*For example, *Nursing Scan in Research: Applications for Clinical Practice* (A NURSECOM Inc. publication) and *Clinical Nursing Research* (a recent journal from Sage Publications, Inc.).

particularly regarding criteria for applicability to a specific setting. For example, it is critical to know the extent to which findings have been replicated and the degree to which risk is involved in application. Two models that outline such criteria have been developed by (1) the well-known CURN group (Horsley et al., 1978) and (2) Stetler and Marram (1976). As mentioned previously, the structured, organizationally oriented CURN model assumes the need for planned change. That of Stetler and Marram is a practitioner-oriented model that assumes research-based information should be part of a critical thinking approach to practice for clinicians, managers, or educators. It thus views utilization broadly and, potentially, pervasively; for example, it is distinguished by the following characteristics (Stetler, 1989; Stetler & Marram, 1976):

- It involves an individual practitioner, *or* a group of practitioners such as the standards committee, *or* the department as a whole.
- It occurs in highly routine, "unplanned" interactions, *or* as part of an ongoing effort to make research findings more visible in day-to-day deliberations and decision making, *or* as a formal introduction and an evaluation of specific findings by means of planned change.
- It results in "indirect" or cognitive applications, *or* one of a variety of "action" applications—for example, as a model for behavior, evidence for change, a catalyst for evaluation, or a component of a complex problem solution.

Such research-based decision making, whether formal or informal, should enhance the scientific base of practice and thereby improve the quality of care, management, or education. As Wyszewianski's work (1988) would suggest, such research utilization should enhance the likelihood that the right thing is done and done "right!" Again, however, the user must be knowledgeable regarding basic research concepts, the process and criteria for research utilization, and the substantive topic of concern.

The second type of research product that can be invaluable to the definition and assessment of quality is the valid reliable measuring tool. In 1984 Lang and Clinton reviewed the assessment of quality of nursing care and, to some extent, the existence of such instruments. Several well-known process tools were cited: QualPac, the Phaneuf audit, and the RUSH-Medicus system (Hegyvary & Haussmann, 1976; Wright, 1984). Of particular note, however, is Ventura's preliminary finding (1980) that such "similar" tools do not necessarily measure the same aspects of process; for example, quality scores on the QualPac, a concurrent tool, did not correlate to any significant degree with quality scores from the Phaneuf audit, a retrospective tool.

Well-researched, general tools on structure and outcomes have not been as readily available as those on process. As Marek (1989) suggests: "Due to the complexity of nursing phenomena, valid and reliable outcome measures are not easily achieved. The majority of current outcome measures have not been tested for validity and reliability" (p. 4). However, with the present emphasis by the Joint Commission and others on outcomes, increasing attention will be paid in both the clinical and the nursing research literature to such instruments. The efforts of the Agency for Health Care Policy and Research (Lang & Marek, 1991; Salive, Mayfield, & Wiessman, 1990), as well as those of the National Center for Nursing Research (ANA, 1990) will be critical in this effort. (See Chapter 4 for further discussion of tools.)

Of importance for this discussion is the potential use of any "ready-made" instruments when the need for measurement of a specific aspect of practice or management arises. Once located—for example, through a computerized journal search or review of reference texts such as those by Waltz and Strickland (1988)—a critical review must be conducted. More specifically, once a potential tool is located, it is important that the nurse manager carefully and critically review its applicability to the quality issue of concern:

1. What needs to be measured? For example, what are your evaluative objectives? Do you want data on process or outcomes? What aspects of process? Do you want self-report or observer ratings?
2. What is the exact purpose of available tools; their level of validity and reliability; the type of data that will result and the analyses required?
3. What is the degree of fit between the tool and the defined need; the cost of collection and analysis; and if copyright is involved, the cost of purchase?

The nurse manager must be a wise consumer and understand what a given tool (e.g., a patient classification or performance evaluation tool) will and will not do for the department. No tool is perfect, but consumers must understand what they need and whether a given instrument can reliably and validly provide a reasonable source of data.

A final research "product" that can influence the quality of care relates to technology. Theoretically, various patient care devices, equipment, or supplies should be marketed on the basis of research results. Such scientific data on product efficacy, however, are not always readily available. Again, with the emphasis on outcomes in health care, this situation may change in the future (Wagner, 1991). At a minimum, it is reasonable to request supportive data from competitive sources of costly and potentially dangerous technologies and to review them critically.

Utilization of research process. The second strategy for enhancing the quality of care and related activities through research utilization involves use of concepts and methods of the research process. In some instances, this strategy resembles or even describes formal evaluative programming (such as the "quality assurance studies" of Kerfoot & Watson, 1985) or formal/pilot change efforts (such as the "action research" of Webb, 1989, or of Hunt, 1987). Before that area of potential confusion and disagreement is addressed, however, other less structured uses of research processes should be considered.

Again, critical thinking and decision-making skills—and thereby quality—can be enhanced through knowledge and use of specific research concepts. Once more, it can occur on both a formal and an informal basis and involves integration of utilization into routine, day-to-day activities. For example, knowledge and application of the concepts of reliability and validity can improve the quality of various data collection efforts within the service setting. Institution-specific audit tools, staff surveys, patient questionnaires, performance appraisal forms, evaluation tools, needs assessments, exit interviews, and so forth, are routinely needed. If no well-developed, relevant tool already exists, then someone within the department probably will be assigned to create one. In doing so, the quality of the data will be enhanced by simply piloting the tool with a few individuals (ANA & Sutherland Associates, 1982); by having a few internal experts systematically review the tool for reliability and content validity; or by constructing a "tabular-form mockup" of outcome data to determine whether the information collected will truly be useful. Such research-related actions, although not at the sophisticated level of methodologic research, may prevent the collection of uninterpretable, inaccurate, or incomplete data.

Other examples of the utilization of components of the research process that may directly or indirectly affect structure, process, or outcome quality include the following:

1. Periodic determination of the reliability of routinely utilized instruments, as for patient classification. This is not necessarily a given component of a classification system, and the validity of the data is thus questionable (Ventura, Hageman, Slakter, & Fox, 1980).
2. Sampling of staff members or patients to obtain needed information. This concept can provide a cost-effective means to collect data (see ANA & Sutherland Associates, 1982).
3. Operational definition of components of a new program, for example, in primary nursing, determining in observable terms what "accountability" means.

Another way in which the research process can be integrated into the service setting is as a model for formal problem solving, evaluation, product evaluation, or quality assessment. It is here where the confusion with research itself is greatest, and, as indicated previously, that confusion is intensified by use of terms such as *quality assurance study, action research,* or *evaluation research.* Even the CURN's organizationally oriented model of "research utilization" (Horsley et al., 1978) adopted for the QAMUR model (Watson et al., 1987) involves such a highly structured and time-consuming approach that it is difficult at times to distinguish it from research itself.

It certainly is true that at times nurse managers need information that is credible only if collected in a highly structured manner within the institution, such as decisions regarding the effectiveness of a controversial model of delivery; the value of a major, costly innovation or change in practice or management; or the acceptability of a recommended product that will represent a sizable capital investment. The same need for credible information, and thus structure, may be required by clinicians to institute a desirable change in practice because of resistance on the part of medical colleagues, limited findings in the literature, or the level of risk involved in the intervention. In such cases, acquisition of theoretic knowledge is not the short-term issue; rather, identification of data that will guide or support a cost-effective decision is required. The research process provides a model for the collection of such data, despite the fact that the intent of data collection is different from that of the conduct of research (Isaac & Michael, 1982; Patton, 1978). The degree of rigor that will be employed will, among other things, depend on issues of cost, immediacy of the need, skill of the problem solvers, level of resistance to change, and even interest in disseminating the project to other institutions through publication.

The dilemma of course is to obtain credible information, but at a reasonable cost. The more rigorous the project, the higher the cost and more than likely the longer the time frame. As Hinshaw and Smeltzer (1987) state, "Research requires a great deal of time. . . . it is not unusual for administrative and clinical studies to involve from 1 year to 2.5 years in the process of investigation" (p. 22). If one accepts the concept of a research-evaluation continuum, theoretically it would be possible to place various program evaluations or quality assurance projects along this continuum. Some would then indeed warrant the title research, whereas others would constitute evaluation (or, in the context of this chapter, research utilization of varying degrees of rigor).

A question could be raised as to whether this focus on terminology is merely one of semantics. In one respect it may not be relevant whether a well-structured, credible project is called research or research utilization or evaluation. On the other hand, the following should be considered:

1. What is the intent of the project? If the key concern is whether the right thing was done and done "right" (Wyszewianski, 1988), the administrator must be certain that the project, whatever it is called, meets the relevant criteria for objectivity and accuracy. If the intent is to evaluate predetermined goals, then the administrator must be certain that the project, again, whatever it is called, meets that criterion to a satisfactory degree. (See Worthen and Sanders [1973, p. 301] for a proposal format for program evaluation in contrast to a research proposal format.)

2. What is the accepted meaning of the term *research* within the agency? Does it connote the "hard" science approach? Is this important to the nursing community? Will nursing's credibility be affected when quality assurance "research" or "studies" are conducted and do not meet the scientific standards of other professionals? If a project is called research, is review by an institutional review board, as well as informed consent, not required?

3. What, if any, constraints are involved in the conduct of a specific, formal, quality-oriented project? If time, money, lack of expertise, and/or lack of control are significant factors, can sufficiently rigorous "research" be conducted to make it credible both within the institution and within the scientific nursing community?

The bottom line is that terminology may indeed make a difference; at a minimum, the nurse administrator must insist that terms be well defined and understood by all involved parties. Perhaps nursing should build on Berwick's terminology (1989) from the field of health services research and use the term *research* to refer only to studies of efficacy (knowing what works) and use *quality assurance* to refer only to the evaluation or study of appropriateness (using what works) and the evaluation or study of the execution of care (doing well what works).

Quality Assurance and Research

The primary focus of this chapter has been on the contribution that research utilization can make to quality improvement. This discussion, however, would not be complete without reference to the reverse relationship, that is, what quality improvement activities can do for research (Grant, Fleming, & Calcarico, 1991; Nadzam, 1991). Quality assurance activities could, of course, identify problems that require basic research exploration. Also, if data have been systematically collected and recorded in a reliable and valid manner, basic theoretic questions could be answered in a cost-efficient manner through secondary analysis (Polit & Hungler, 1991). With the advent of computerized nursing information systems, large data bases could routinely become available to nurse researchers. With appropriate planning, research and quality assurance/improvement could truly become formally integrated (Grasso & Epstein, 1989).

ADMINISTRATIVE IMPLICATIONS

Nurse administrators are responsible for ensuring the quality of nursing care provided within their setting. The role that research can play in that process has been identified in the following terms:

1. The development of knowledge that can form the scientific basis for practice and/or management by means of the *conduct* of research in order to determine the "right thing"

2. The application of such scientifically acquired knowledge and/or related tools, products, or processes by means of the *utilization* of research in order to enhance implementation of the right thing in the right way

The nurse administrator must consciously decide how each of these strategies fits with the goals of the nursing organization and related issues of quality. Projects that take the form of formal research normally will require a considerable amount of time. Their potential impact on quality thus will be long-term but could benefit patients beyond the study setting. For administrators with limited resources, but a strong desire to institute such research projects, collaborative arrangements with a university may provide an attractive strategy.

For issues of quality in the here-and-now, research utilization provides more immediate impact. It offers flexibility and potential influence on a widespread, integrative basis. It also can enhance formal activities in an established program of quality assurance.

Whichever approach to the integration of research and quality is chosen, the skills of various levels of personnel must be addressed. Studies indicate that a high level of research knowledge cannot be assumed to exist (Stetler & Sheridan, 1988; Thomas & Price, 1984). The same is more than likely true for knowledge of research utilization (Stetler, 1989; Stetler & DiMaggio, 1991). Persons who are expected either to conduct or to use research must already be knowledgeable, be provided with continuing education, or be given adequate systems of support (research/utilization consultation). In turn, individuals with the requisite preparation (clinical nurse specialists or master's-prepared nurse managers) must be expected to explicitly demonstrate incorporation of research relative to their responsibilities in the assurance of quality.

CONCLUSION

Nursing research and quality of nursing care do have an explicit relationship. It is, however, one that will not occur by chance, and its exploration is a major challenge for today's nursing service administrator.

REFERENCES

American Nurses' Association Council of Nurse Researchers. (1990). NCNR update, *CNR, 17,* 1.

American Nurses' Association and Sutherland Learning Associates, Inc. (1982). *Nursing quality assurance management learning systems: Guide for nursing quality assurance coordinators and administrators.* Kansas City, MO: American Nurses' Association.

American Nurses' Association Task Force. (1988). *Standards for organized nursing services and responsibilities of nurse administrators across all settings.* Kansas City, MO: Author.

Berwick, D. (1989). Health services research and quality of care: Assignments for the 1990s. *Medical Care, 27,* 763-771.

Beyers, M. (1988). Quality: The banner of the 1980s. *Nursing Clinics of North America, 23,* 617-623.

Bloch, D. (1980). Interrelated issues in evaluation and evaluation research: A researcher's perspective. *Nursing Research, 29,* 69-73.

Brett, J. (1987). Use of nursing practice research findings. *Nursing Research, 36,* 344-349.

Briones, T., & Bruya, M. (1990). The professional imperative: Research utilization in the search for scientifically based nursing practice. *Focus on Critical Care, 17,* 78-81.

Coyle, L., & Sokop, A. (1990). Innovation adoption behavior among nurses. *Nursing Research, 39,* 176-180.

Cronenwett, L. (1987). Research utilization in a practice setting. *Journal of Nursing Administration, 17*(7, 8), 9-10.

Gaits, V., Ford, R. N., Kaplow, R., Bru, G., Belcher, A., Brown, S., & Bookbinder, M. I. (1989). Unit-based research forums: A model for the clinical nurse specialist to promote clinical research. *Clinical Nurse Specialist, 3,* 60-65.

Goode, C., Lovett, M., Hayes, J., & Butcher, L. (1987). Use of research based knowledge in clinical practice. *Journal of Nursing Administration, 17*(12), 11-18.

Grant, M., Fleming, I., & Calcarico, A. (1991). Research and quality assurance. In M. Mateo & K. Kirchhoff (Eds.), *Conducting and using nursing research.* Baltimore: Williams & Wilkins.

Grasso, A., & Epstein, I. (1989). The Boysville experiment: Integrating practice decision-making, program evaluation, and management information. *Computers in Human Services, 4,* 85-94.

Haller, K., Reynolds, M., & Horsley, J. (1979). Developing research-based innovation protocols: Process, criteria and issues. *Research in Nursing and Health, 2,* 45-51.

Hefferin, E., Horsley, J., & Ventura, M. (1982). Promoting research-based nursing: The nurse administrator's role. *Journal of Nursing Administration, 12*(5), 34-41.

Hegyvary, S., & Haussmann, R. (1976). Monitoring nursing care quality. *Journal of Nursing Administration, 6*(9), 3-9.

Hinshaw, A., & Smeltzer, C. (1987). Research challenges and programs for practice settings. *Journal of Nursing Administration, 17*(7, 8), 20-26.

Hoare, K., & Earenfight, J. (1986). Unit-based research in a service setting. *Journal of Nursing Administration, 16*(4), 35-39.

Holzemer, W. (1980). Research and evaluation: An overview. *Quality Review Bulletin, 6,* 31-34.

Horsley, J., Crane, J., & Bingle, J. (1978). Research utilization as an organizational process. *Journal of Nursing Administration, 8*(17), 4-6.

Horsley, J., Crane, J., Crabtree, M., & Wood, D. (1983). *Using research to improve nursing practice: A guide (CURN project).* New York: Grune & Stratton.

Hunt, M. (1987). The process of translating research findings into nursing practice. *Journal of Advanced Nursing, 12,* 101-110.

Issac, S., & Michael, W. (1982). *Handbook in research and evaluation.* San Diego: EDITS Publishers.

Kerfoot, K., & Watson, C. (1985). Research-based quality assurance: The key to excellence in nursing. In J. McCloskey & H. Grace (Eds.), *Current issues in nursing* (2nd ed.). Oxford: Blackwell Scientific Publications.

Kerlinger, F. (1964). *Foundations of behavioral research.* New York: Holt, Rinehart & Winston.

Kirchhoff, K. (1982). A diffusion survey of coronary precautions. *Nursing Research, 31,* 196-201.

Lang, N., & Clinton, J. (1984). Assessment of quality of nursing care. *Annual Review of Nursing Research, 2,* 135-163.

Lang, N., & Marek, K. (1991). The policy and politics of patient outcomes. *Journal of Nursing Quality Assurance, 5*(2), 7-12.

Larson, E. (1983). Combining nursing quality assurance and research programs. *Journal of Nursing Administration, 13*(11), 32-35.

Leape, L. (1990). Practice guidelines and standards: An overview. *Quality Review Bulletin, 16,* 42-49.

Lieske, A. (1985). Quality assurance and research. In C. Meisenheimer (Ed.), *Quality assurance: A complete guide to effective programs.* Rockville, MD: Aspen Publications.

Lindquist, R., Brauer, D., Lekander, B., & Foster, K. (1990). Research utilization: Practical considerations for applying research to nursing practice. *Focus on Critical Care, 17,* 342-347.

Luker, K. (1981). An overview of evaluation research in nursing. *Journal of Advanced Nursing, 6,* 87-93.

Marchette, L. (1985). Developing a productive nursing research program in a clinical institution. *Journal of Nursing Administration, 15*(3), 25-30.

Marek, K. (1989). Outcome measurement in nursing. *Journal of Nursing Quality Assurance, 4*(1), 1-9.

Nadzam, D. (1991). The agenda for change: Update on indicator development and possible implications for the nursing profession. *Journal of Nursing Quality Assurance, 5*(2), 18-22.

Patterson, C. (1988). Standards of patient care: The Joint Commission focus on nursing quality assurance. *Nursing Clinics of North America, 23,* 624-638.

Patton, M. (1978). *Utilization-focused evaluation.* Beverly Hills, CA: Sage Publications.

Peters, D., & Pearlson, J. (1989). Clinical evaluation: Research or quality assurance. *Journal of Nursing Quality Assurance, 3*(3), 1-6.

Polit, D., & Hungler, B. (1991). *Nursing research: Principles and methods* (4th ed.). Philadelphia: J. B. Lippincott.

Reeves, D., Underly, N., & Beckwith, B. (1982). Establishing a research subcommittee in a service institution. *Nursing and Health Care, 3,* 189-192.

Rizzuto, C., & Mitchell, M. (1988). Research in service settings. I. Consortium project outcomes. *Journal of Nursing Administration, 18*(2), 32-37.

Sahney, V., Durkewych, J., & Schramm, W. (1989). Quality improvement process: the foundation for excellence in health care. *Journal of the Society for Health Systems, 1,* 17-29.

Salive, M., Mayfield, J., & Wiessman, M. (1990). Patient outcomes research and the Agency for Health Care Policy and Research. *Health Services Research, 25,* 697-708.

Scogna, D. (1981). Nursing research in a cancer cooperative group setting. *Cancer Nursing, 4,* 277-280.

Staff. (1990). Can research change the way MDs practice medicine? *Hospitals,* October 5, 32-38.

Stetler, C. (1984). *Nursing research in the service setting.* Reston, VA: Reston Publishing Co.

Stetler, C. (1985). Research utilization: Defining the concept. *IMAGE: Journal of Nursing Scholarship, 17,* 40-44.

Stetler, C. (1989). A strategy for teaching research utilization. *Nurse Educator, 13*(3), 17-20.

Stetler, C., & DiMaggio, G. (1991). Research utilization among clinical nurse specialists. *Clinical Nurse Specialist, 5,* 151-155.

Stetler, C., Marram, G. (1976). Evaluating research findings for applicability in practice. *Nursing Outlook, 24,* 559-563.

Stetler, C., & Sheridan, E. (1988). Measuring knowledge of consumerism. In O. Strickland & C. Waltz (Eds.), *Measurement of nursing outcomes* (Vol. 2). New York: Springer.

Stokes, J. (1981). Utilization of research findings by staff nurses. In S. Krampitz & N. Pavlovich (Eds.), *Readings for nursing research.* St. Louis: C. V. Mosby.

Thomas, B., & Price, M. (1984). *Thomas-Price inventory of nursing research: Instructor's manual.* St. Louis: C. V. Mosby.

Van Servellen, G. M., & Stetler, C. (1986). Utilization of research: Critiquing research for practice. In A.M. Lieske (Ed.), *Clinical nursing research.* Rockville, MD: Aspen Systems.

Ventura, M. (1980). Correlation between the quality patient care scale and the Phaneuf audit. *International Journal of Nursing Studies, 17,* 155-162.

Ventura, M., Hageman, P., Slakter, M., & Fox, R. (1980). Interrater reliabilities for two measures of nursing care quality. *Research in Nursing and Health, 7,* 25-31.

Wagner, M. (1991). Outcomes research affecting devices. *Modern Healthcare, 21*(6), 54.

Waltz, C., & Strickland, O. (1988). *The measurement of nursing outcomes: Vol. 1. Measuring client outcomes.* New York: Springer.

Watson, C., Bulecheck, G., & McCloskey, J. (1987). QAMUR: A quality assurance model using research. *Journal of Nursing Quality Assurance, 2*(1), 21-27.

Webb, C. (1989). Action research: Philosophy, methods and personal experiences. *Journal of Advanced Nursing, 14,* 403-410.

Weiss, C. (1972). *Evaluation research: Methods of assessing program effectiveness.* Englewood Cliffs, NJ: Prentice-Hall.

Wiese, R. (1989, October). Key aspects of comfort conference participants 6 months later. *Nursing Research Nursing Practice: Connection,* p. 6.

Woody, M. (1980). An evaluator's perspective. *Nursing Research, 29,* 74-77.

Worthen, B., & Sanders, J. (1973). *Educational evaluation: Theory and practice.* Belmont, CA: Charles A. Jones.

Wright, D. (1984). An introduction to the evaluation of nursing care: A review of the literature. *Journal of Advanced Nursing, 9,* 457-467.

Wyszewianski, L. (1988). Quality of care: Past achievements and future challenges. *Inquiry, 25,* 13-22.

CHAPTER 14

Educational Preparation
for Quality

Marilyn T. Molen

The problems facing nursing education today are a reflection of issues that affect both the health care industry and the educational system in the United States. The nurse of the future is the one who is able to act and reflect with a mind that never ceases to inquire or expand. Education for quality means preparing a compassionate scholar-clinician for practice in a dynamic, ever-changing, health care environment.

More than 10 years ago, Mary Kelly Mullane (1977) made a statement at a deans' seminar sponsored by the American Association of Colleges of Nursing (AACN) that still rings true today: "I believe so strongly that in times of stress we have a special need to review roots, our history, our purposes, our priorities. Only in that way can we determine with intelligence and care what changes are appropriate and in the best interest of all concerned."

Nursing is in a time of acute stress, and the problems facing nursing education are a reflection of issues that affect both the health care industry and the educational system in the United States. In confronting these issues, nursing must consider not only the current situation and the forces leading to it but also the directions that most likely will lead us to a positive future. In the words of Schlotfeldt (1985, p. 244), "Nurses

Metropolitan State University, 121 Metro Square, St. Paul, MN 55101.

Series on Nursing Administration — Volume III, 1992

themselves must create a new and improved future appropriate for the challenges that lie ahead for their future."

Educating for quality means, first of all, that we must know what kind of practitioner is needed and for what kind of practice. Our educational programs must then be structured and methodologies developed to meet those needs. If we do not respond to this challenge, professional nurses will be inadequately prepared for our desired future.

ISSUES AND CHALLENGES

The health care industry is facing a crisis because of the shortage of nurses. To delineate the factors contributing to this shortage, the DHHS Secretary's Commission on Nursing issued an interim report in 1988. Findings indicated that the current shortage is primarily a result of an increase in demand rather than a contraction of supply: "The Commission is concerned that the shortage of RNs is affecting quality of patient care, the work environment for RNs, and access to health services" (p. 7). The testimony provided by witnesses appearing before the Commission and the written statements submitted in response to invitations for comments, as well as recent studies and reports, all point to a growing concern regarding the negative consequences of the current shortage on the practice of nursing.

Furthermore, the Commission reported that nursing's future is not particularly optimistic in view of a predicted demand for registered nurses that will continue to increase without a commensurate increase in supply. The challenge of educating for quality means addressing the issue of quantity, that is, providing adequate training to a sufficient number of workers to meet the health care system demands. It also means preparing the type of professional practitioner who can adjust to a dynamic and rapidly changing health care system.

Changes in the health care system have been forced by the continued explosion of knowledge and technology and the rapid advancement of information and communication systems. If predicted changes in these areas continue, our traditional approaches to teaching and learning will not offer adequate preparation for professional nursing practice. In projecting some specific changes in health care, Ginzberg (1987) predicted that hospitals would lose between 10% and 15% of their current job complement (400,000 to 600,000 positions) over the next 10 years. During this period, convalescence services would experience the greatest growth, particularly in home health care services in which an additional 500,000 to 800,000 jobs will be created. Approximately 20% to 30% of these jobs will be medically related to include positions for nursing, therapy, and related personnel. Ginzberg also predicted rapid growth in ambulatory care settings, with 825,000 to 1,050,000 more jobs created over the next 10 years (Bezold & Carlson, 1986).

Ginzberg's prediction for registered nurses is that the supply will increase, but employment opportunities will shift from hospitals to out-patient and home care services. He believes that nurses prepared at the postbaccalaureate level will be in greater demand as supervisors and for work in high-tech units. The better-prepared nurses will have greater flexibility in shifting between clinical and administrative roles. Personnel at the lower skill levels, such as the assistants and technicians, will experience job obsolescence because automation will take over their current responsibilities. Nursing homes, home health care, and other modalities of care, especially for elderly and chronically ill persons, will become major sources of employment. Summarizing from major govern-mental forecasts for nursing (including those of Ginzberg), Bezold and Carlson (1986) report that 50% to 80% of the primary treatment modal-ities can be handled by protocols. In support of their assertion, they cite a listing of typical complaints screened by health maintenance organiza-tions. Of these complaints, 63% were handled through protocols. Health care personnel, especially nurses, will have to adjust to software proto-cols and related therapeutic delivery technologies in their practice.

Styles and Holzemer (1986) report that, based on current trends, by the year 2000 there will be about half the number of nurses trained at the baccalaureate and higher-degree levels as needed. They predict an over-supply of 501,000 technical (associate degree and practical) nurses in contrast with a shortage of 619,000 professional (baccalaureate and higher degree) nurses by the turn of the century. To achieve goals for the future, the authors suggest an educational remapping by adjusting down-ward the preparation of technical nursing personnel and adjusting up-ward the preparation of professional nursing personnel. "Professional nurses provide greater flexibility for the system; they act more knowl-edgeably in complex environments and more autonomously in isolated environments. Also extended care facilities and home health care increas-ingly require substantial clinical judgments as well as planning and tech-nical skills" (Styles & Holzemer, 1986, p. 66). To accomplish this remap-ping, the authors suggest strategies that include (1) discontinuing all nursing education programs in noncollegiate settings, (2) merging the practical and associate degree nursing programs for an overall reduction in technical personnel, and (3) doubling the number of graduates from baccalaureate programs by increasing the enrollments in existing generic and second-step programs and by establishing new programs in locations where the need is great and the resources for high-quality programs are available.

Aydelotte (1987) predicts that over the next 25 years, both nurses and the health care system in which they work will be quite different. Con-tinued development of biotechnology will be accompanied by new legal and ethical concerns. Artificial intelligence will lead to more sophisti-cated clinical and administrative decision making. Health care economics will raise serious questions of social ethics and governmental responsibility for both access to health care and allocation of health care resources. Aydelotte agrees that the knowledge base required for practice will be extensive, regardless of the type of practice or its setting. She describes the practice of nursing in the future as consisting of several functions, including "surveillance, diagnostic reasoning, provision of personal needs, and the care of the environment" (p. 118). Nursing also will consist of several roles such as "the assurance of personal interaction, support for coping and refreshing, and education of individuals on how to use programs and technology, including machines and telematics" (p. 118).

Detmer (1986) reiterates several of these points in her predictions of the future in health care. She calls for well-prepared and experienced nurses to provide the observations and appropriate livesaving interventions as acuity levels of hospitalized patients increase. Unfortunately, she also predicts that the already insufficient role of the nurse in promoting health and self-care instruction for inpatients will diminish and fall to the nurse in the ambulatory setting because of time constraints. She stresses the importance of nurse-to-nurse communication as patients move in and out of health care systems with care responsibilities delegated to others, including the patient's family. Home care, Detmer believes, offers exciting opportunities for nursing in promoting teamwork and coordination of services in a cost-effective manner. The current movement toward managed care and case management in nursing suggests that these may be ways of achieving the intended outcome.

To achieve our desired future in nursing, Aydelotte proposes several strategies, most of which are directed toward educational preparation for quality. Pointing out that a profession must reflect a knowledge base that is unique, she says we must strive to clarify and understand the nature of our profession to achieve a knowledge base exclusive to nursing. She argues that nursing has been too preoccupied with numbers. We should develop a cadre of professional nurses with intelligence and motivation who are mature and capable of self-regulation. These professional nurses need a sound educational foundation to achieve excellence in clinical practice and administration.

SETTING THE EDUCATIONAL DIRECTIONS

The public is well aware of the concern that has been raised over the quality of education from the grade school through the postsecondary levels. Summarizing the current status of educational reform, a statement in a local newspaper announced that "attention now is focused on such things as how teachers do their jobs, who makes school decisions, and whether schools are educating students to meet the challenges of the future" ("State's schools," 1988, p. 1B). As a result of these reform efforts, Aydelotte predicts that by the year 2010, "individuals will be educated, more informed, and more highly skilled in the use of information available to them" (p. 114).

Indicating the level of concern over quality of education in the United States, Sakalys and Watson (1985) reported that six significant studies conducted during the 1982-1985 period all found serious problems in American education. From each study came similar recommendations for improving the quality of education, from the primary through the post-secondary and professional levels. The common recommendations were categorized into three areas: curricular, instructional, and administrative.

The curricular recommendations were (1) to restore the centrality of the liberal arts at all educational levels, (2) to increase the structure and coherence of curricula, (3) to emphasize intellectual skills such as problem solving, and analytic and critical thinking, (4) to emphasize mastery of basic principles rather than specific facts, (5) to emphasize fundamental attitudes and values, (6) to emphasize lifelong learning, (7) to decrease specialization at the baccalaureate level, and (8) to emphasize a broad and rigorous baccalaureate education as the basis for professional preparation.

Recommendations in the instructional area were (1) to increase the emphasis on "good teaching," (2) to emphasize active modes of learning, (3) to increase the use of Socratic teaching strategies and promote faculty development in this methodology, and (4) to promote student-faculty interaction within the learning situation.

Recommendations for the administrative area were (1) to promote leadership and support for educational rigor and reform, (2) to revise the reward system in promoting high-quality instruction, (3) to promote faculty development in effective teaching and instructional strategies, and (4) to increase support for educational research.

In carrying out efforts at educational reform and change, Felton (1987) sounds a warning about the dilemma of having to reconcile the two countervailing forces that seem to exist between the goal of excellence and quality on the one hand and the goal of opportunity and equity on the other. She reminds us that higher education must keep its sights on the system's objective, which is "to provide citizens with as much education as they are willing to seek and are capable to achieving" (p. 126). In resolving these distinctions, Felton suggests that the most important issues in nursing education may not be between professional and liberal, or even between general and special but, instead, between serious and trivial and between responsible and irresponsible. Quality education, she asserts, "has to do with institutions defining what an educated person is rather than letting people define it for themselves" (p. 127).

Schlotfeldt (1985) shares this view in promoting the development of autonomous professional schools of nursing. She observes that "organized nursing, to date, has been singularly unsuccessful in instituting an educational system through which to prepare and award credentials to practitioners who are uniformly competent, at least at a minimal acceptable level, to practice as independent, general practitioners of professional nursing. It is the leaders in the profession, notably those in academia, who are in a position to correct those deficiencies" (p. 247).

Measures of Educational Quality

The concept of educational quality often is elusive, with varying meanings, ranging from a mystical view that defies measurement to an assessment of quality according to outcomes of the educational processes. To measure quality, it must first be defined. Cornell (1985) offers a quality assurance definition of the term: "Quality assurance involves assuring the consumer of a specified degree of excellence through continuous measurement and evaluation of structural components, goal-directed process, and/or outcomes, using pre-established criteria and available standard norms, followed by appropriate alterations with the purpose of improvement" (p. 356). This definition describes the recent emphasis on the "value-added" approach to assessing educational quality. Focus on educational outcomes, or the value added as a result of the educational process, is seen as an appropriate response to the criticisms of higher education posed by declining enrollments, accelerating inflation, and the declining status of education within the national priorities.

Although the value-added method has gained widespread popularity, it is only one of several approaches to assessing educational quality. Four of the most common ways of determining quality have been through mystique, reputation, resources, and outcomes (Cornell, 1985). Although mystique cannot be measured, it has been used by some as a way of judging the quality of an educational program. When reputation is used to evaluate educational quality, it involves both process and product. The assessment considers students, faculty, and administrators, as well as degrees, honors, and research activities. Resources sometimes are used to judge the quality of a program on the assumption that environmental factors affect the student and the educational process. This form of quality assessment overlaps with reputation as a quality indicator. Those who favor using outcomes to measure educational quality argue that "true quality resides in the institution's ability to affect students favorably and to make a positive difference in their intellectual and personal development" (Cornell, 1985, p. 357). The value-added method of measuring educational outcomes "includes collection and analysis of objective and subjective data on the students so that a baseline can be established and gains can be determined through repeated data collection. By determining the relative changes in one student or in a cohort of students, the impact of the specific program or total university can be assessed" (Cornell, 1985, p. 357).

The indicators of quality for professional nursing education have been specified in great detail. Rogers (1985), for example, suggests the following basic requirements: (1) a comprehensive college or university, (2) an organizational structure for nursing, (3) a qualified nursing faculty, (4) lower-division general education and appropriate upper-division cognate courses in the arts and sciences, (5) a substantive upper-division major in nursing characterized by the transmission of an organized body of scientific nursing knowledge, (6) laboratory study whereby students have an opportunity to translate theoretic knowledge in nursing into human service directed toward maintaining and promoting health and caring for and rehabilitating the sick and disabled, (7) instruction in how to exploit nursing knowledge for the improvement of the practice of nursing, (8) acculturation of the student as a learned professional—as a peer of other professional personnel, and (9) development of personal and professional accountability and responsible citizenship.

When new and existing programs are evaluated, the common indicators used to judge their quality generally include the qualifications of the faculty and students and the program of study and the resources available to it, as well as the administration and evaluation of the program ("Position statement," 1987).

Assessment of Quality in Nursing Education

The criteria for professional accreditation delineate specific requirements that must be met to ensure that minimum standards of educational quality have been achieved. The criteria for the evaluation of baccalaureate and higher-degree programs in nursing have been categorized according to the following program components: (1) structure and governance, (2) material resources, (3) students, (4) faculty, (5) curriculum, and (6) evaluation (Council of Baccalaureate and Higher Degree Programs [CBHDP], 1988). These components will serve as the organizing framework for the assessment of quality in nursing education that follows.

Structure and Governance

The academic system, which has developed as a collegial system over centuries, is giving way to the formal structure of business and to hierarchical decision making. The corporate trend seen in other organizational structures is making its way into colleges and universities. As Hechenberger (1988) points out, "for the first time in at least 30 years, schools of nursing must respond to environmental conditions in a buyer's market rather than a seller's market" (p. 281). She urges that a good dose of "corporate" discipline be imposed upon the academy. It has been observed, however, that as a corporate group of functionaries, nurses and leaders in nursing have given mixed messages about their eagerness, and even willingness, to participate in this brave new world. Schlotfeldt (1985) exhorts scholars and professionals prepared at the highest levels to provide the kind of leadership that will ensure continued progress in each discipline and profession, as well as in society at large. Nursing, she believes, has deprived itself of that assurance because of corporate nursing's failure to opt for an appropriate future. She cites an urgent need for schools of nursing to become fully autonomous by having complete control over their entire educational enterprise.

Within a very competitive environment, schools of nursing are highly vulnerable unless they understand the importance of strategic planning, marketing and public relations, fiscal responsibility, and fund raising. Administrators of schools that survive will have made these areas their number one priority. According to Hechenberger (1988), nursing needs strong leadership that is willing to adjust pragmatically to these changing times. Administrators must undertake strategic planning that outlines how the nursing program extends the mission of the university and provides a unique contribution to the educational effort. They must be able to provide data outlining measures of cost effectiveness, along with plans to generate new dollars. Some schools will survive this era of constraint; others will not. The closing of the school of nursing at Boston University illustrates the gravity of the situation. As Hechenberger (1988) points out, "From now on the administration of these programs will reflect a more conscious effort to plan the course of their development, to relate process to outcome, and to seek an optimal return both quantitatively and qualitatively from limited resources" (p. 281).

A study of five top-ranked schools of nursing was conducted in 1985 to determine their organizational climate as models of excellence to be emulated in attracting top faculty, students, and funding (Haussler, 1988). From these top five schools, 180 faculty completed an organizational climate index questionnaire. Data from this survey were compared with data from an earlier survey of six baccalaureate nursing programs in the New England area. Findings showed that faculty in the top-ranked schools of nursing perceived a greater degree of freedom for individual expression and less organizational restrictiveness on their behavior. There also seemed to be less focus on procedural orderliness and conformity to a defined norm of personal appearance and institutional image. A rather surprising finding was that faculty in three of the top-ranked schools believed there was less support. This may have been, in part, because the heavy demands for research, advanced degrees, and other service activities left little time for social and collegial relationships.

In emulating these top schools of nursing, Haussler encourages an environment that promotes high standards of achievement with few constraints on individual expression. She urges us to avoid procedures that block creativity and personal freedom and directs us to provide support based on the maturity of individual faculty members so that they will have both the freedom and the responsibility to do their jobs as they see fit.

Material Resources

Quality education depends on adequate resources to meet the needs of the program. These include computer services, library resources, laboratory access to clinical facilities, and financial and other institutional resources judged necessary to support both program and students' needs ("Position statement," 1987). Reflecting the importance of these support services was a report in *The Chronicle of Higher Education* indicating that many prospective students now measure the quality of a college or university by the availability of computers on its campus. To students this is "an indicator of an institution's financial health, its commitment to student services, and its modernity" (DeLoughry, 1988, p. A1).

Nursing education draws heavily upon the resources of an institution. In 1987 a study costing out baccalaureate nursing education was conducted by Arthur Young for the Division of Nursing, Bureau of Health Professions, DHHS (Kummer, Bednash, & Redman, 1987). Findings from this study indicated that the average cost of preparing one nurse at the baccalaureate level in 1986-1987 was $51,000. According to this report, the total cost of generic baccalaureate nursing education in the United States during the 1983-1984 period was approximately $1 billion dollars. Analysis of both direct (nursing) and indirect (nonnursing) instructional costs indicated that they amounted to approximately 2.9% of the expenditures for all instruction at 4-year institutions in the United States. Of the 970,000 baccalaureate degrees awarded in all disciplines during this period, generic nursing degrees composed approximately 2.5% of the total.

A study of generic baccalaureate program trends was conducted by Redman, Cassells, and Jackson (1985) in 1984. Participating in this survey were 246 deans drawn from the AACN membership list. Among the findings from this study was the report that most deans believed that their schools were either well or adequately funded and that they were receiving higher or equal priority for funding than were other programs at their universities. Two thirds of the respondents thought most of their support services were adequate.

Yet another study of the fiscal status of nursing educational programs in the United States indicated that budgeting for these programs was becoming more difficult (Gunne, 1985); 82% of these respondents reported this opinion, although most nursing deans still believed they were getting their fair share. Of those responding 23% indicated that budgetary constraints had resulted in some reformulation of their program objectives. Even so, 55% said they expected program quality to remain the same, although 23% thought quality would increase and 21% thought it would decrease. As the competition for scarce resources increases, nurse administrators will have to exercise prioritization and reallocation in order to maintain program quality. As Hechenberger (1988) points out: "In addition, declining enrollments, deteriorating facilities, smaller state appropriations, fewer federal dollars, and more competition for private dollars imply a different approach to the recruitment, retention, and graduation of nursing students and to the overall administration and governance of schools of nursing" (p. 281).

It is encouraging to note that the deans of baccalaureate programs, as a whole, believe they are keeping up with competition from other programs (Cassells, Redman, Haux, & Jackson, 1988). In a recent follow-up survey of AACN programs (N = 453), 90% of the deans perceived their funding at the same level or higher than the funding of other programs. In comparing their 1986-1987 budgets with the previous year, the majority (53%) reported a higher budget, although 19% indicated their budgets were lower. The three resources found to be most adequate were audiovisual equipment, library collections, and office space for faculty and administrators. Computer resources also were considered good.

Students

As recently as 1984, deans of baccalaureate programs were reporting that their schools were maintaining or increasing enrollments and attracting a significant number of students who already held baccalaureate or higher degrees in other fields (Redman et al., 1985). Since that time the downward turn has been dramatic. Analysis of a 10-year trend, between 1977 and 1986, showed an overall decrease of 10.4%. During the previous decade, baccalaureate admissions dropped 6%, associate degree admissions rose 5.6%, and diploma admissions plummeted 56% (Rosenfeld, 1988).

Even more discouraging is evidence that the decline in numbers of nursing aspirants has been accompanied by a decline in the academic ability of those who are pursuing nursing careers. Data from a survey of 300,000 college freshmen at nearly 600 institutions support this assertion (Green, 1987). Results from this 1986 study show that the Scholastic Aptitude Test (SAT) scores of high school students interested in nursing are well below the national average. Furthermore, SAT scores of prospective nursing students have been declining so that the gap between nursing and nonnursing aspirants has widened. Farrell (1988) reports that figures from the College Board totaled 689 for nursing applicants in 1986. This score was 217 points below the SAT average, and a gap of 177 points existed between nursing and nonnursing applicants. Grade-point average data are consistent with this finding. The freshman survey data also indicated that a larger proportion of the nurses—almost one third— had C+/C grade-point averages than did nonnurses.

Findings from the aforementioned survey show migration of academically able women from nursing to other fields. As Ginzberg (1987) points out, "The critical point about women in the labor market is the vast opening of opportunities" (p. 1596). He reports that the majority of all new entrants into the accounting field are women. Almost half (40%) of the new entrants in law are women, and 35% of the new admissions to medical school are women. American colleges are now awarding approximately 16,000 medical degrees in contrast to some 14,500 baccalaureate nursing degrees (Green, 1987).

Even more discouraging, the Cooperative Interinstitutional Research Program (CIRP) data (Green, 1987) show that more than half (52.4%) of the college freshman women who initially chose nursing changed their plans during their undergraduate years. According to this report, the attrition rate for nursing students is higher than that of most entering freshmen. One factor that seems to contribute to this out-migration is the structured nature of nursing programs. A longitudinal study of nursing students who entered college in 1982 and who were resurveyed in 1986 indicated that "one of the most important predictors of persistence in nursing was essentially a characteristic often called the authoritarian personality: the people who stayed in nursing were the people who liked very structured areas. Those who left were those who could not handle the high level of structure" (Green, 1987, p. 1612).

The pool of candidates for nursing has been changing in other ways. Over 20 years of data from the CIRP project show substantial shifts in attitudes, values, and goals of American college students. According to these findings the transition in life goals has been from "developing a meaningful philosophy of life" to "being very well-off financially" (Green, 1987, p. 1610). The demographics also show a change in the age cohort. With a decline in the 18- to 24-year-old applicant pool, it is projected that the number of college students older than 25 years of age will continue to increase.

Enrollment shifts have occurred in most nursing programs. The proportion of RN students and part-time students has increased in baccalaureate programs. Despite this increase in the RN student population, overall admissions and enrollments continued to decline. Aiken (1987) predicts that "the number of nursing graduates is expected to drop from a high of almost 83,000 in 1985 to approximately 68,000 by 1995" (p. 1616). Others have said that baccalaureate enrollments will have to double to achieve the desired numbers of professional nurses needed by the turn of the century (Naylor & Sherman, 1987). Overall, the demographic projections of the supply of health workers are not encouraging. As the CIRP study shows, with the 15% to 20% decline in college-aged students over the past decade, even if the proportion of persons pursuing health careers remains the same, the numbers will still decrease (Green, 1987).

In light of these grim statistics, 392 AACN schools were contacted in the spring of 1987 to determine the strategies that have been used to attract and retain quality students (Naylor & Sherman, 1987), and 58% of the schools (N = 226) responded to the survey. Findings show that, in general, schools of nursing were just beginning marketing and recruitment efforts to counteract the decline in quality and quantity of the applicant pool. Of the marketing strategies reported by the deans of these schools, among the most effective have been (1) personal contact with faculty, students, and alumni (N = 141), (2) open house and career days (N = 86), (3) visits to high school counselors (N = 74), (4) visits to hospitals and community colleges (N = 72), (5) brochures and printed advertisements (N = 68), and (6) college career fairs (N = 54).

Innovative program options have been particularly helpful in recruiting RN students to baccalaureate programs. Among those listed in this report were (1) flexible scheduling of classes during evenings, on weekends, or during summer session, (2) special tracts for RN students, and (3) accelerated program options. With the changing student demographics, ways must be found to accommodate a student body that is characterized by its heterogeneity. We need to be more flexible in our curriculum planning so that all students are not forced to progress through the same program.

Naylor and Sherman (1987) suggest a comprehensive solution to the present nursing dilemma: "The success of strategies to attract the best and the brightest to nursing will be measured, in large part, by our success in restructuring the professional work environment and in changing the public negative image of nursing" (p. 1603). They recommend that strategies include "creating nursing markets; maximizing the opportunities for reimbursement of nursing services; creating growth opportunities for nursing professionals, developing an educational system to attract the brightest and best, and assuring optimal federal and state support for nursing."

Aiken (1987) also advocates restructuring the practice environment so that it can operate more effectively with fewer nurses. Given the declining enrollments, she believes that the ultimate solution to the nursing shortage may be fewer, better-paid nurses. She suggests specific strategies, including (1) more support staff and technical assistance, such as computers and word processors, for nurses and (2) more career ladder options, along with the rewards and status that will keep nurses at the bedside. Ginzberg (1987) gives implicit support to this general approach by agreeing that to have more and better nurses is a sound idea, but he raises the critical question, "Who will pay?"

Naylor and Sherman's proposed comprehensive solution (1987) has begun to have some positive results. For instance, the Robert Wood Foundation and Pew Charitable Trust, Inc., have invested more than $25 million in a national program to strengthen hospital nursing. The program is directed toward restructuring the health care system to promote higher quality, more cost-effective care. Eighty hospitals and/or consortia across the nation were involved in planning grants in 1989-1990. Of these, 20 were recipients of $1 million to implement their plans for strengthening hospital nursing over the next 5 years. The outcome of this program should be a major redesign of the workplace, with nursing in a pivotal role.

In response to the steady decline in the number of students selecting nursing as a career, the Governing Board of the National Committee on Nursing Implementation and the Advertising Council of New York are coordinating a 3-year public service campaign to improve the image of nursing and to attract more men and women into the profession. The result of this successful effort was a 5.9% increase in 1989-1990 that snapped the 5-year enrollment decline in nursing (AACN, 1991). Comparisons between a 1990-1991 survey conducted by the AACN and one conducted the previous year indicate that enrollment rose by another 10.6%. Nevertheless, although these encouraging signs are welcome, other conditions are likely to prolong the nursing shortage well into this decade. According to AACN (1991, p. 7), "2,292 prospective, qualified bachelor's degree students were turned away in the current 1990-91 academic year by nursing programs that did not have sufficient resources to accommodate them." Increasing the supply of nurses also has been slowed by the popularity of part-time study, which delays the rate of graduates entering the health care system.

In addition to these national programs, other strategies for recruitment to nursing have been proposed and some have been tested. At Beth Israel Hospital, for instance, a pilot program called "choose nursing" has been initiated in partnership with a local school. Through this program, eleventh-grade students have been identified to learn more about nursing. The goal of this program is to offer fellowships for interested students to pursue a nursing career (Cushman & Warnick, 1987).

Farrell (1988) and Felton (1987) both recommended that, rather than yielding to the temptation of lowering admission requirements, we reach out more fully to our minority population. Farrell argues persuasively on behalf of minority student recruitment by citing the need for health professionals who are culturally aware and sensitive to the particular needs and concerns of different ethnic groups. With the population shifts occurring in our society, it seems appropriate to adjust recruiting strategies, as well as curricular emphases, to meet changing multicultural needs.

Although previous efforts to attract minorities had limited success, it is encouraging to note that recent efforts are beginning to show some improvements in the statistics. The 1990-1991 AACN survey results indicate that a significant proportion of first-time nursing students pursuing baccalaureate degrees (17.1%) are members of a racial or an ethnic minority group: "Of these, Blacks represent the largest number (10.6%) followed by Asians (3.2%), Hispanics (2.8%) and Native Americans (0.5%)" (p. 7). Native Americans are still severely underrepresented in nursing programs.

One of the primary reasons cited by AACN deans for the declining enrollments has been the decreased financial support for students, along with the increased tuition and other financial charges within the educational setting (Naylor & Sherman, 1987). In response to fiscal constraints, a number of recommendations for tuition reimbursement, as well as loans and scholarships, have been forwarded at the local, state, and federal levels. One of these proposals has been targeted at disadvantaged high school students as an untapped pool to recruit for nursing. In 1988 Senator Edward Kennedy (D, MA) proposed a bill (HR 4648) calling for a "partnership" arrangement that would provide a 25% federal grant and a 75% loan to eligible students interested in pursuing nursing careers. The grant would cover tuition, books, child care, and living expenses. After graduation, the graduate would work in a sponsoring hospital or nursing home that would pay back two thirds of the loan. The remainder of the loan would be paid back by the graduate over a 2- to 4-year period (Staff, 1988).

Innovative approaches to ease the financial burden of nursing students can be found in various settings. According to the *New York Times* (Hevesi, 1988), one hospital in Chicago has been willing to pay tuition, not only for their nurses but for their spouses and children as well.

In a number of states, nursing coalitions have been formed to help address the nursing shortage and to enhance the image of nursing. In Minnesota, for example, a coalition of statewide nursing organizations called the Council of Minnesota Nursing Organizations (CMNO) was established to speak with one voice on issues affecting nursing and to promote a positive future for nursing. This organization is addressing several issues, especially those related to differentiated practice and educational articulation. A related coalition, called the Coalition on Nursing, is comprised of CMNO representatives, as well as representatives of the local and statewide organizations of hospital administrators. This coalition is focusing more specifically on the issues of nursing recruitment and retention in the hospital arena.

Faculty

The faculty of an educational program is a key element in determining the quality of that program. Illustrating this point in a dramatic way is a report that nursing colleges in the Philippines have been suffering a "severe brain drain" as faculty members have left for the United States in search of higher pay (Cohen, 1988). This report indicates that all the nursing programs in the Philippines are now short of qualified faculty, and as a consequence, they no longer are able to maintain their educational standards. Because of the declining quality of nursing education, fewer than half of the 5000 to 7000 graduates from these nursing colleges passed the licensing examination in 1988.

It is no wonder then that appointment, retention, and development of well-qualified faculty are of major concern to the academic administration of an educational institution. To ensure educational quality, the number of faculty members and their academic and experiential backgrounds must be sufficient and diverse enough to meet the goals of the nursing program. Faculty members must have proper credentials and must demonstrate competence in their areas of instructional responsibility. The level of faculty preparation must be appropriate to meet the goals of the program. The program must have a faculty that demonstrates expertise in the areas of curriculum, instruction, and research. In addition to effectiveness in teaching, program quality depends on faculty endeavors that include scholarly activities, professional activities, and community service (Council of Baccalaureate and Higher Degree Programs, 1983 and 1988).

To maintain the standards for professional accreditation, nursing programs must provide evidence that the aforementioned requirements have been met. The AACN survey of baccalaureate nursing education (Cassells et al., 1988) provides a demographic profile of faculty in nursing education programs that is different from that of faculty, as a whole, in colleges and universities. The *Chronicle of Higher Education Almanac* (1988) indicates that the proportion of women faculty members at public and private institutions is approximately 28%. In contrast, the proportion of women faculty members in nursing programs is approximately 98%. As recently as 1988, the majority of faculty members teaching in baccalaureate programs still held a master's degree (75.1%) as their highest level of educational preparation. In the AACN survey (Cassells et al., 1988), 20.5% reported holding a doctorate, and 5.9% were prepared at the baccalaureate level only. In an earlier AACN report (Redman & Jackson, 1987), a comparison of the percentage of doctorate-holding faculty in baccalaureate programs since the first survey was conducted in 1978-1979 shows an increase in the proportion of nursing faculty with doctorate degrees from 15.0% that year to 31.8% in 1986-1987. This finding represents a steady increase in the educational level of faculty over 9 consecutive years. A similar comparison of mean faculty salaries and percentage of change by rank and doctoral preparation between 1985-1986 and 1986-1987 shows increases ranging from 4.3% to 9.2%. Despite this positive finding, it is well known that faculty salaries in general have not kept pace with the cost of living.

Cassells et al. (1988) report that 46% of the responding deans indicated that their institutions had a tenure track. "The mean percent of tenured faculty teaching on the baccalaureate level was 38% (N = 321), with a range from 1% to 100% of the nursing faculty" (p. 44). This finding is considerably below the national figures, which show that the proportion of faculty with tenure at public institutions is 68.9% and at private institutions is 54.7% (*Chronicle,* 1988). During the past 10 to 15 years, mainstreaming of nursing faculties into the promotion/tenure system of colleges and universities has occurred. In general, they are now expected to comply with the same stringent criteria as those established for all faculty in academia. Thus nursing faculties are meeting the same demands for excellence in teaching, scholarly productivity, and service as their academic counterparts in other university departments. Centers of research and other faculty development efforts have been instituted to support faculty members in their efforts to expand the knowledge base of nursing and to meet the promotion/tenure requirements of the university. In the 1988 AACN survey, deans reported that full-time faculty members in baccalaureate programs receive an average of 3.28 days a month for professional development, which is defined as research, writing, continuing education, and conferences (Cassells et al., 1988).

With the recent proliferation of doctoral programs in schools of nursing, the demands on faculty as scholars and leaders are even greater. Indicators of quality in these programs reflect a higher level of expectation for active engagement in research and knowledge development that are theoretically and philosophically relevant to the phenomena of nursing. This includes publication of research and scholarly activity in journals that are subject to peer review. Faculty members are expected to serve as mentors to students in initiating them into a career-oriented and scholarly focus, and they are expected to facilitate a community of scholars among students and their peers ("Position statement," 1987). In this milieu, it is not surprising that "nursing faculties will need to work differently, better, more systematically, and most likely, longer and harder to fulfill the tripartite mission of teaching, research, and community service" (Hechenberger, 1988, p. 281).

Curriculum

Assessment of educational quality must take into account three components of the curriculum: (1) the theoretic knowledge base that determines the structure and design of the curriculum, (2) curricular content or subject matter, and (3) instructional methodologies used to achieve goals of the program. Each of these areas is discussed in the sections that follow.

Knowledge base. Rogers (1985) describes the distinguishing characteristics of professional education in nursing as "the transmission of nursing's body of abstract knowledge, arrived at by scientific research and logical analysis — not a body of technical skills" (p. 381). It is this organized body of theoretic knowledge that defines the profession of nursing. The process of education includes not only the transmission of this theoretic core of knowledge but also the acquisition of skills of practice and the inculcation of a set of professional values.

Professional nursing education provides a foundation of principles that are drawn from nursing, the sciences, and the arts and humanities, which constitutes the knowledge base from which critical judgments in practice are drawn. Nursing has a social mandate to demonstrate a unique critical mass of knowledge, which is identified as the discipline of nursing. Although the distinct body of knowledge is essential for the preparation of professional nurses, Schlotfeldt (1987) asserts that a point of consensus on this matter has yet to be reached by a cadre of professionals in the field. Issues pertaining to the mission and goals of nursing, as well as its domain and focus, must be resolved in order to be clear about our image as a profession and our roles and functions in nursing practice. Many of the unresolved issues in practice, Schlotfeldt contends, reflect unresolved issues in the system of education.

One of the factors that contributes to the inconsistencies in the educational system has been nursing's vacillation between two higher educational models, the academic model and the professional model (Forni & Welch, 1987). The academic model emphasizes a strong liberal arts base from which study in the discipline follows. The professional model tends to introduce students to the discipline at a relatively early stage while offering coursework that directly supports study in the profession. The importance of selecting one model or the other, or developing a new model, is that it creates an image for the discipline. Resolving this issue would help strengthen nursing as a respected discipline.

Nursing has matured in its ability to establish the critical mass of knowledge for the discipline. Several factors are now in place to do this. Today nursing has scholars and research organizations, as well as other resources and services that can be used in launching a major effort to carry out the type and amount of scholarly effort that are needed to make a substantial contribution to the development of a knowledge base for nursing (Stevenson, 1988).

Another important step toward resolving some of the educational issues surrounding the preparation of nurses for professional practice is the evolution of recommendations from the AACN-sponsored study of the essentials of education for professional nursing (AACN, 1987). The panel that conducted this study has recommended that every program that prepares nurses for professional practice include educational experiences that are considered essential. The educational components identified as essential are (1) the context of nursing and its effect on education, (2) socialization within the profession, (3) liberal education, (4) values and professional behaviors, and (5) professional knowledge and nursing practice. These essential components should be used in establishing the structure and design of the curriculum, in determining the subject matter to be emphasized, and in planning and implementing teaching methodologies.

Regardless of substance and structure, most agree that a nursing curriculum must promote the skill of critical thinking. In addition to the knowledge and skill they possess, nurses must be able to make critical judgments and lifesaving decisions in their practice. They are required to solve complex problems and to think critically in their daily work. To evaluate the role of education in promoting critical thinking, Tiessen (1987) conducted a study in a large Midwest baccalaureate nursing program to determine which of eight selected variables had contributed most to students' ability to think critically. Results of this study showed that about one fourth (24%) of the variance of nursing students' critical thinking ability was associated with a cluster of variables, which included SAT quantitative scores, grade-point average, and total number of credit hours in the arts and humanities. The findings indicated that students' ability in mathematics correlated most strongly with their skill in critical thinking. From these results, Tiessen recommends that SAT scores, both verbal and mathematics, be given careful consideration in the decisions regarding student admission. She also recommends that mathematics proficiency be monitored and, if necessary, remediation efforts instituted to ensure that graduates can function adequately in the practice setting.

One nursing program has already instituted a remedial program for students identified as academically at risk. To facilitate successful completion of their program requirements, the Clemson University College of Nursing has established a Nursing Resource Center (Hughes, 1988). At-risk students are identified by screening their records according to three criteria: (1) grade-point average less than 2.0 at the end of the sophomore year, (2) academic probation at the end of any semester, and (3) one or more D grades in any nursing course. All students who qualify for assistance through the center are followed through the remainder of their program to graduation. Services provided through the center include individual counseling, tutorial assistance, and referral to other campus sources as needed.

The correlation between credit hours accumulated in the arts and humanities and students' analytic ability, found in Tiessen's study (1987), offers support to the importance given to the liberal arts component of professional nursing education. Liberal education is intended to help students in solving problems, in gathering and sifting information, and in making decisions. It also helps develop the qualities of the mind that help the person to live a more full and satisfying life. Inasmuch as a major function of nursing is to enhance the well-being of others, nurses need to have an educational base that will enable them to foster well-being and continued growth (AACN, 1987). Although the actual content of liberal education generally is conveyed through the arts, humanities, and social sciences, the spirit of liberal education should be emphasized in all courses. The student as the central part of the educational process and excellence in teaching are essential components of a liberal education (Newell, 1985).

Socialization, values, and professional behaviors also are essential elements of professional nursing education. Although socialization is largely a subconscious process, it is the means by which the student develops a sense of identification with and commitment to the profession. Through the process of socialization, a member of the profession internalizes the values and norms of that profession. Faculty members play an important role in facilitating the socialization process through role modeling, demonstrating mastery of the knowledge, skill, and other attributes of the profession, and conveying a commitment to the values and obligations of the profession. These socialization strategies should be included as part of the educational process. Similarly, the development of values, attitudes, and behaviors that characterize members of the profession should be fostered throughout the curriculum (AACN, 1987).

Curricular content. Subject matter in the curriculum is directed by the philosophy and conceptual framework of the program. It also is influenced by societal changes that affect professional practice. "Rapid changes in health care, especially those related to age groups, care settings and technology, require that the professional nurse have an up-to-date knowledge and practice base, the motivation and skills for lifelong learning, and the ability to translate new knowledge and skills into health care for individuals, families, groups, and communities. These changes have implications for curricular content, clinical learning sites, new areas of specialized knowledge, and changed responsibilities" (AACN, 1987, pp. 54-55).

In a survey of AACN deans (Redman et al., 1985), the majority of the respondents indicated that several trends could influence curriculum planning over the next decade. Among those listed were ambulatory, outpatient, and home care rather than hospital care; proactive participation in formulating health care policy; health education of consumers; contractual agreements with corporations for the provision of nursing services; increased numbers of independent nurse practitioners; and establishment of stress management programs and centers. In response to these trends, deans reported that some schools had begun to emphasize health promotion and health maintenance, leadership and management skills, community health with a home health focus, gerontology, computerization, and preceptorship experiences. Many deans reported increased collaboration with clinical agencies, along with many perceived benefits.

In the follow-up AACN survey (Cassells et al., 1988), deans indicated that the two most important educational goals now are (1) to provide an awareness of comprehensive health care and (2) to develop the intellectual and creative capabilities of the learner. They identified changing health needs, advances in the science and practice of nursing, and evolving economic and political circumstances as major factors influencing the curriculum. Areas of particular interest and concern included ethical issues and dilemmas in nursing practice, computer technology, gerontology, long-term care, cross-cultural nursing, and the AIDS epidemic.

Illustrating the curricular response to a changing health care scene, the proposed master's degree program in nursing at Metropolitan State University in the Twin Cities has been designed to help shift the paradigm of nursing practice from an occupation to a profession. Upon admission, students will select a high-risk population in need of professional nursing knowledge and skill. Their mentors throughout the program will be experts in the practice setting. Their practice will be directed toward managing the care of clients in this high-risk population. A portfolio of coursework applications to this high-risk population will be developed systematically through the curricular sequence. Students will have intensive internships with their practice mentors. A final project will allow them to test the fiscal and health outcomes of their professional practice with the high-risk population. From this educational preparation, it is expected that each graduate will be able to demonstrate, through the portfolio review, a model of professional practice for a selected high-risk population.

Teaching methodologies. Instructional strategies must be adequate to meet the needs of the program. They also must keep pace with changes that are occurring in the education of health professionals. In her State of the School of Nursing address, Dean Rhetaugh G. Dumas (1988) predicted that "the focus of education for the health disciplines will be on problem solving, critical thinking, and analytical skills. Students will assume more responsibility for their own learning. Teachers will spend less time on lectures and will utilize information/communications technologies more extensively in assisting students to locate and retrieve information from computer-stored data" (p. 3). Computer technology will be used to help students become proficient in clinical decision making and in patient care. Computers will replace the traditional form used for evaluation. Dumas warns that traditional approaches to teaching and learning will be rendered obsolete by the turn of the century.

To cope with the frustration of trying to prepare generalists for a highly specialized health care system, Billue (1988) advocates an approach that emphasizes lifelong learning. She views learning as a continuous effort that must be integrated into the student's life-style as are diet and exercise. To teach students to value learning as a form of personal growth, she advocates a focus on the affective domain. Good communication and role modeling help motivate students. Active participation in the learning process also fosters attitude development. Learning strategies such as discussion, independent projects, and practice/application experiences can be used to reinforce active learning.

In brief, the curriculum must prepare professional nurses with knowledge and with the cognitive and critical thinking skills that will encompass the care of individuals, families, groups, and communities in a variety of settings. The educational process must encourage socialization into the nursing profession and the instillation of values and behaviors that are consistent with the profession.

Evaluation. The criteria for accreditation of baccalaureate and higher-degree programs in nursing specify that "the findings from the ongoing systematic evaluation of all program components are used for program development, maintenance and revision" (CBHDP, 1983, p. 9). Because the need for careful program planning has never been more important, it is essential to have an adequate data base that will provide sufficient qualitative and quantitative information to use in establishing priorities and allocating resources. An evaluation plan that is well conceived and truly operational provides the base for program modification and strategic planning that will be essential for the survival of nursing education in today's competitive environment.

CONCLUSION: TOWARD THE FUTURE

Recognizing the challenge that lies ahead, nursing education currently is promoting workshops and conferences that will set new directions for curriculum development and teaching. Illustrating this effort was a workshop sponsored by the National League for Nursing in 1988. This workshop was designed to introduce faculty members to some basic theoretic constructs underlying a new curriculum paradigm and to assist them in developing teaching strategies that will support a new future for nursing. The programming of this workshop reflects a belief that graduates of today's educational programs must be "those who can accept the ambiguities of the modern medical and health care world—a complex world—in which there are no certainties nor any easy and clear solutions and everyday judgments are fraught with ethical and moral dilemmas that require daily reevaluation of our most basic ideas about human life" (Bevis & Watson, 1988). The objectives of this program were directed toward (1) helping faculty perceive a different role for the teacher, along with a different set of responsibilities, (2) examining the criteria for methodologies that will move the learner forward on the learning continuum so that the desired skill, professionalism, meanings, patterns, and insights might be achieved, and (3) developing criteria for the selection of student-faculty interactions that will foster growth and liberation of the student and that rely on trust and criticism rather than on testing.

As Bevis and Watson (1988) point out, the nurse of the future is the one who is able to act and reflect with a mind that never ceases to inquire or expand. Educating for quality means preparing a compassionate scholar-clinician for practice in a dynamic, ever-changing health care environment. The challenge is here before us. Let us meet it with vision and with vigor.

REFERENCES

Aiken, L. (1987). Breaking the shortage cycles. *American Journal of Nursing, 87,* 1616-1620.

American Association of Colleges of Nursing. (1987). Essentials of college and university education for professional nursing. *Journal of Professional Nursing, 3,* 54-71.

American Association of Colleges of Nursing. (1991). Students being turned away from nursing schools. *Legislative Network for Nurses, 8*(2), 7-8.

Aydelotte, M. K. (1987). Nursing's preferred future. *Nursing Outlook, 35*(3), 114-120.

Bevis, E., & Watson, J. (1988). *New directions of a new age: Curriculum development for professional nursing education.* Unpublished manuscript.

Bezold, C., & Carlson, R. (1986). Nursing in the 21st century: An introduction. *Journal of Professional Nursing, 2,* 2-9.

Billue, J. S. (1988). Life-long learning: An answer to the content controversy. *Journal of Professional Nursing, 4,* 241, 308-309.

Cassells, J. M., Redman, B. K., Haux, S. C., & Jackson, S. S. (1988). RN baccalaureate nursing education. 1986-1988 (Research Grant No. DIO NU 23072). Washington, DC: Department of Health and Human Services.

Chronicle of Higher Education Almanac. (1988, September 1), p. 3.

Cohen, M. (1988). Nursing colleges in Philippines suffer doubly as both teachers and students seek foreign jobs. *The Chronicle of Higher Education,* p. A24.

Cornell, G. R. (1985). The value-added approach to the measurement of educational quality. *Journal of Professional Nursing, 1,* 356-363.

Council of Baccalaureate and Higher Degree Programs. (1983). *Criteria for the evaluation of baccalaureate and higher degree programs in nursing* (Publication No. 15-1251A). New York: National League for Nursing.

Council of Baccalaureate and Higher Degree Programs. (1988). *Criteria for the evaluation of baccalaureate and higher degree programs in nursing.* Working draft.

Cushman, M., & Warnick, M. (1987). Searching for excellence. *American Journal of Nursing, 87,* 1638-1642.

DeLoughry, T. J. (1988). Once they asked: How many library books? Now it's: Are computers available at 3 a.m.? *The Chronicle of Higher Education, 25*(3), A1, A38.

Department of Health and Human Services, Secretary's Commission on Nursing. (1988, July). Interim report. Washington, DC: Author.

Detmer, S. S. (1986). The future of health care delivery systems and settings. *Journal of Professional Nursing, 2,* 20-27.

Dumas, R. G. (1988, Spring). From the dean. In *Notes and News,* University of Michigan School of Nursing.

Farrell, J. (1988). The changing pool of candidates for nursing. *Journal of Professional Nursing, 4,* 145, 230.

Felton, G. (1987). Obstacles to nursing's preferred future. *Nursing Outlook, 35*(3), 126-128.

Forni, P. R., & Welch, M. J. (1987). The professional versus the academic model: A dilemma for nursing education. *Journal of Professional Nursing, 3,* 291-297.

Ginzberg, E. (1987). Facing the facts and figures. *American Journal of Nursing, 87,* 1596-1600.

Green, K. (1987). What the freshmen tell us. *American Journal of Nursing, 87,* 1610-1615.

Gunne, G. M. (1985). The fiscal status of nursing education programs in the United States. *Journal of Professional Nursing, 1,* 336-347.

Haussler, S. (1988). Faculty perceptions of the organizational climate in selected top-ranked schools of nursing. *Journal of Professional Nursing, 4,* 274-278.

Hechenberger, N. B. (1988). The future of nursing education administration. *Journal of Professional Nursing, 4,* 279-284.

Hevesi, D. (1988, July 31). Shortage of nurses forces a rise in salaries. *New York Times,* pp. 1, 16.

Hughes, R. B. (1988). The nursing resource center: Facilitating academic success. *Journal of Professional Nursing, 4,* 289-293.

Kummer, K., Bednash, G., & Redman, B. (1987). Cost model for baccalaureate nursing education. *Journal of Professional Nursing, 3,* 176-185.

Mullane, M. K. (1977). Nature of the university or college: Mission of the nursing unit. Paper presented at the American Association of Colleges of Nursing deans' seminar, Sun Valley, ID.

Naylor, M. D., & Sherman, M. B. (1987). Wanted: The best and the brightest. *American Journal of Nursing, 87,* 1601-1605.

Newell, L. J. (1985). Shall the twain meet? Liberal education and nursing education. *Journal of Professional Nursing, 1,* 253-254.

Position statement. (1987). Endorsed by AACN, October, 1986. Indicators of quality in doctoral programs in nursing. *Journal of Professional Nursing, 3,* 72-74.

Redman, B. K., Cassells, J. M., & Jackson, S. S. (1985). Generic baccalaureate nursing programs: Survey of enrollment, administrative structure/funding, faculty teaching/practice roles, and selected curriculum trends. *Journal of Professional Nursing, 1,* 369-380.

Redman, B. K., & Jackson, S. S. (1987). *Report on nursing faculty salaries in colleges and universities.* Washington, DC: American Association of Colleges of Nursing.

Rogers, M. E. (1985). The nature and characteristics of professional education for nursing. *Journal of Professional Nursing, 1,* 381-383.

Rosenfeld, P. (1988). *Nursing student census with policy implications* (Publication No. 19-2202). New York: National League for Nursing.

Sakalys, J. A., & Watson, J. (1985). New directions for higher education: A review of trends. *Journal of Professional Nursing, 1,* 293-299.

Schlotfeldt, R. M. (1985). A brave new nursing world: Exercising options for the future. *Journal of Professional Nursing, 1,* 244-251.

Schlotfeldt, R. M. (1987). Resolution of issues: An imperative for creating nursing's future. *Journal of Professional Nursing, 3,* 136-142.

Staff. (1988). Congress eyes an education "partnership." *American Journal of Nursing, 88,* 1270.

State's schools to offer choices, changes. (1988, September 5). *Star Tribune,* p. 1B.

Stevenson, J. S. (1988). Nursing knowledge development. *Journal of Professional Nursing, 4,* 152-162.

Styles, M. M., & Holzemer, W. L. (1986). Educational remapping for a responsible future. *Journal of Professional Nursing, 2,* 64-67.

Tiessen, J. B. (1987). Critical thinking and selected correlates among baccalaureate nursing students. *Journal of Professional Nursing, 3,* 118-123.

Index

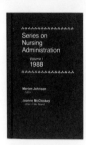
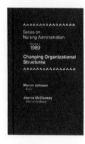